Lisa Fitzpatrick

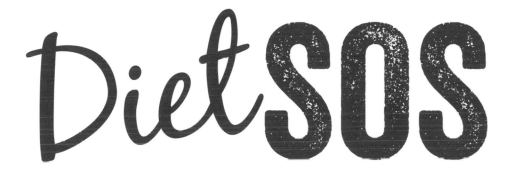

DietSOS

Life changing tips for long-term weight loss success

K

Thank you...

Shonagh Lyons – Thank you for your dedication and hard work throughout this whole process. Your enthusiasm made this journey exciting and fun. Here's to working on many more projects together because you are a joy to work with.

Noel Kelly at NK Management – Thank you for your constant support, advice and most of all friendship. You know me so well and always encourage me to challenge myself. x

Niamh Kirwan at NK Management – I feel as if I never work a day in my life when working with you. You make my job easy. You are always positive and a wonderful sounding board. You are a great friend. x

Judith Hannam – Thank you for your guidance and support over the last year. It has been a real pleasure to work with you. x

First published in Great Britain in 2014 by
Kyle Books, an imprint of Kyle Cathie Ltd
192–8 Vauxhall Bridge Road
London SW1V 1DX
general.enquiries@kylebooks.com
www.kylebooks.com

10 9 8 7 6 5 4 3 2 1

ISBN 978 085783 172 9

Text © 2014 Lisa Fitzpatrick
Design © 2014 Kyle Books
Photographs © 2014 Tara Fisher *
Illustrations © 2014 Tim Weiffenbach

* except pages: 43: ©iStock.com/stphillips; 85: ©iStock.com/elenathewise;
88: ©iStock.com/iwhiteout

Lisa Fitzpatrick is hereby identified as the author of this work in accordance with Section 77 of the Copyright, Designs and Patents Act 1988.

A Cataloguing in Publication record for this title is available from the British Library.

Editor: Judith Hannam
Editorial Assistant: Claire Rogers
Copy Editor: Catherine Ward
Designer: Heidi Baker
Photographer: Tara Fisher
Food and props stylist: Annie Rigg
Illustrator: Tim Weiffenbach
Production: David Hearn/Nic Jones

Colour reproduction by ALTA London
Printed and bound in China by 1010 Printing Group Ltd

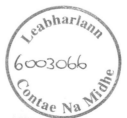

Contents

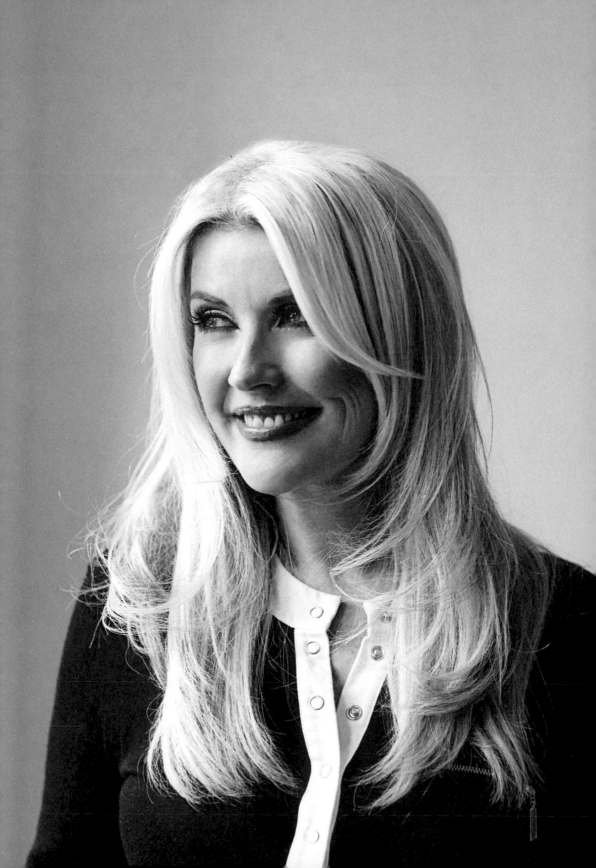

From the very moment I decided to lose weight my life changed. Not dramatically, but it did change. I had reached a point where I could no longer pretend that my weight wasn't an issue. Having Sophie, my first child, gave me the courage I needed to make that change. In her I found my motivation and my incentive to be healthy, and from that point onwards I took control of something that had haunted me for years.

First and foremost, I learned that I was the only person who had the power to do something about my situation. Before that an alien could have dropped down from Mars and said, 'Lisa, for the sake of planet Earth, please lose weight,' and I would still have carried on with my chocolate, chips and bad habits. The point is that the life-changing decision had to come from me – otherwise it would never have worked.

At my heaviest, I was a size 20, weighing around 15 stone. I want to share my personal weight-loss journey with you, as I really believe that what worked for me could work for you. However, before you read any further here are a few home truths I think you should know:

1. Losing weight is not rocket science.
2. There is no quick fix.
3. You are what you consume.
4. Feeling sorry for yourself is a waste of time and will not make you slim.
5. Only you have the power to change.

Let me put my cards firmly on the table: I'm not a diet expert, I'm not a fitness guru, and I'm not a psychologist. I'm a real woman, who was really overweight and who managed to lose those pounds without losing her sanity! I'm a positive thinker and I pride myself on being a good wife, mum and friend.

I love my job as a fashion stylist. However, while I have discovered every trick of the trade when it comes to covering up lumps and bumps, I also recognise that hiding never solved anything – I should know, I owned more oversized cardigans than you'd ever think possible! Covering up might be helpful in the short term, but it certainly isn't the answer.

Deep down, if you know you are truly overweight, there comes a time when you have to take control. Believe me when I say I stumbled more than once, but also believe in yourself and recognise that you are capable of doing this. Just go for it!

Lisa xxx

Chapter one

Identifying THE PROBLEM

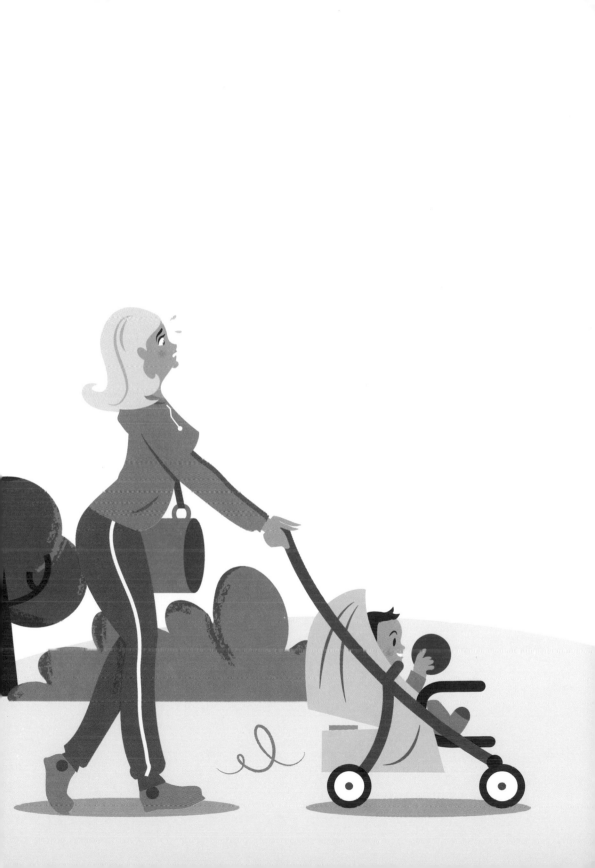

I was brought up in a typical Irish household on big dinners.

My childhood years

I was brought up in a typical Irish household on big dinners consisting of meat and two veg – stews, mince, roasts, that sort of thing. If it was traditional we ate it! And when I say ate I really mean ate. You didn't put your knife and fork down until your plate was empty and only then could you go outside to play. I usually ate fast. It was hearty food and we had regular meals, three times a day. We had cereal for breakfast and the bread was white. Lunch was sandwiches and a packet of crisps. It wasn't always healthy, but it was certainly consistent. When dinner was made at home we used a full bag of potatoes and thought nothing of it. In those days, food was more about fuel and habit than anything else.

Like most children I never really listened to my body when I was younger. I just kept on eating until the food was gone. I didn't really know when I was full because I never gave myself the chance to find out. I certainly never gave any thought to the choices I made in relation to food and that probably paved the way for eating the wrong things as I got older.

Luckily for me I was very sporty, so even though I wasn't eating particularly well my weight was never an issue. I enjoyed exercise and I loved being active. It was something I focused on and I liked the feeling of being fit. I was slim, outgoing and I had a big personality. I always made sure I got my point across! I definitely ate a lot more than I should have done – I found it hard to resist a sugar craving and I rarely deprived myself – but I was so energetic it never seemed to matter. If I wanted it, I ate it! Back then my life was quite simple – it was all about fresh air and fitness.

My teenage years

As a teenager I was tall and slim, with brown curly hair and freckles I wished would disappear. In spite of that I was a happy, outgoing and upbeat girl. I was always on the go and I loved a challenge. When I was in school I did a milk and paper round. At 16 I got my first job in retail, working in our local supermarket. At 17 I worked in a coffee shop and at 18 I went to the United States to be a lifeguard for the summer. I was always independent and enjoyed the responsibilty I had, working from a young age.

I was aware of the importance of good posture and always held myself well – it just seemed natural to me – but I never remember being conscious of my weight at that time. I knew that looks were important to some people, and I seemed to realise quite early on that making the most of your assets was an art form, but while I didn't like my brown hair and wished for bigger boobs I learnt to be content with what I had been given. To me, I dressed well, looked the part and talked the talk. The 80s was a time to have fun with fashion and there was definitely more of an 'anything goes' attitude back then than there is now. There simply wasn't the emphasis on looks and appearance we see today in the media. We didn't have the same culture of being fascinated by celebrities, how they looked and how thin they were. As far as I was concerned, people came in all different shapes and sizes and the most glamorous thing on TV was the annual Rose of Tralee competition, which was all about finding a young woman with a great personality who could become a good ambassador for Ireland around the world. The girls spent some time chatting to the host and then often performed an Irish song or dance as a party piece. I loved it! It just seemed to be a far more innocent time and I don't think women compared themselves to others in the way they do now.

It's fair to say I have always been a people watcher – I could sit all day in a coffee shop and watch those around me – but even though I spent hours doing it, I never found myself being jealous or envious of other women. It just wasn't something that ever occurred to me – I was brought up to be proud of who I was and to believe in myself.

I didn't go to college after I left school. Instead, I went on to do a fitness course and train as an instructor for a year. Somewhere in the back of my mind I didn't consider this to be 'real' study as such and therefore I often felt inadequate when the conversation turned to education in a social situation. I'm not sure why I thought like that because in every other way I had an inner strength I was proud of. It never stopped me from wanting to be successful, it was just something that

> *To me, I dressed well, looked the part and talked the talk.*

The harsh reality was that between the ages of 25 and 30 I gained 5 stone.

made me slightly uncomfortable. As time went on that inadequate feeling did stay with me and it was certainly a factor in my weight gain. It stands to reason that our insecurities can sometimes get the better of us. Food has always been a source of comfort for me, even if the ill-effects of overindulging didn't show straight away.

My early twenties

I fell into the world of women's retail and I was certainly swept away by it. I started out working in retail, followed by wholesale, and I loved everything about the industry. My job took me to different places and I thrived on meeting new people. I knew I was good at it and that made me even more determined. I was fascinated by how women dressed and styled themselves. It opened my eyes to so many new experiences and cultures.

When I was 25, I weighed 9 stone and wore a size 8–10. Thankfully, youth was still on my side and I was lucky with my figure at that point – I was still quite active and had a quick metabolism. Around this time I met my future husband Paul. As clichéd as it might sound, I fell head over heels in love. I had never understood that kind of love before, knowing someone cared for you that much. Being with Paul gave me an increased air of confidence and I loved loving him back. He is certainly my soulmate. As our relationship developed fairly quickly, so did my relationship with food. Suddenly we were eating out three or four nights a week and for the rest we lived on takeaways. It felt like I was discovering food for the first time. It became so much more than a necessity; it had a social aspect that wasn't there before.

The comfort years

As my social life took off my attitude towards eating began to change and food started to become much more than a necessity. By now Paul and I were eating out in different restaurants, tasting new foods and drinking wine. We were both working hard and we thoroughly enjoyed that period of our lives. In fact, I wouldn't have changed it for the world.

When we were at home it was all about comfort – takeaways, our couch, the TV: it was my idea of bliss. The fact that food now played a bigger part in my life seemed only natural. What wasn't natural was that by the time I turned 28 I had gained 2 stone and was wearing a size 14. And, yet, I don't remember being overly worried about my weight at this stage. My life was very busy and I didn't have time to stop and think too much. It might sound strange that I didn't really notice the weight gain myself, but it was definitely obvious to people around me. The problem was there was no let up in the lifestyle we were living. By now our relationship with food had become a worrying habit. The harsh reality was that between the ages of 25 and 30 I gained 5 stone. At 30 I was wearing a size 18–20.

Learning the art of disguise

Before I sat down to write this book I somehow managed to convince myself that even when I was overweight I was happy. But I was deceiving myself. I now know that, as well as hiding my weight, I was hiding how I truly felt. I always had my hair blow-dried, my make-up was perfect and big earrings were my trademark. I invested in shoes, handbags and scarves. To this day many people say they don't remember me that size. The truth is I became a real master at concealing my weight. I wore a one-buttoned, three-quarter length designer coat that I bought in a sale for the best part of three years. It covered everything and felt like my cloak of armour. Once I had it on, I felt like my body was completely hidden and that nobody could see it. Looking back, it is clear I was uncomfortable with how I looked, but all that concerned me at the time was keeping up the illusion. Of course, all the warning signs were there; I just chose to ignore them. I remember the overwhelming feeling of nearly passing out from the heat because I was so covered up, and how I had to use really strong deodorant to cope with the perspiration. Sometimes the heat was so unbearable it felt like I was going through the menopause – often when we were in a bar or a restaurant I'd have to go outside just to feel fresh air and be able to breathe properly! Looking back, it was clear I was nervous about how I felt, looked and spoke. I felt inadeqate in so many ways. It wasn't me – the young confident woman who had a wonderful boyfriend and a great job. My weight had begun to control areas of my life; it was becoming my every thought.

In truth I wasn't happy. Even though I may not have been able to admit it at the time my body had made me incredibly insecure. I was anxious and I was uncomfortable. Everything that I was eating was adding to the problem. I can't

My old diet

Here is an example of what I used to eat in a typical day. Most days I was consuming up to 5000 calories!

8am: Croissant or scone and toast with tea
9am: Breakfast roll with bacon, sausage, egg and ketchup
11am: Tea and chocolate bar or biscuits
12pm: Tea and half a packet of biscuits
1pm: Roll, bag of crisps, chocolate bar
3pm: Tea and biscuits
6pm: Three-course meal with wine/rum and cola

stress enough how the weight gain happened slowly and how I didn't really acknowledge it until it was too late and the damage was done. Not only was I overweight, but I was also unhealthy. I went from being a young girl in her twenties who wore a size 8 to someone who struggled to find clothes for her size.

Looking back, I find it hard to understand why I didn't do something about my weight gain sooner, but the truth is food was an addiction for me, a cycle I didn't know how to break. There were many moments during that time that should have been defining, that should have made me take note, and yet they didn't. Until I decided I needed to lose weight it really was irrelevant what other people said to me.

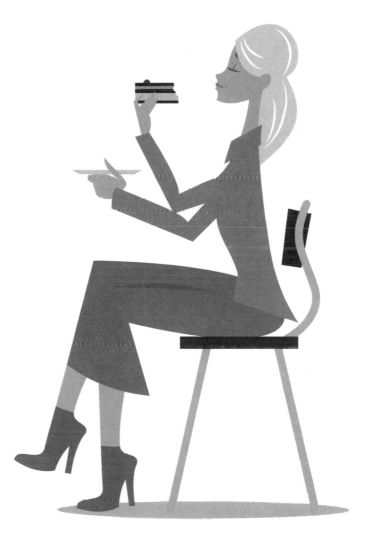

All those diets ever did was focus my mind on what I was not supposed to do.

The diet years

At various times over those years I tried every diet possible. I bought all the books – I tried no carbs, protein only, with carbs: you name it, I did it. If there was a newspaper article about dieting I cut it out and kept it. I read about every new diet and, yet, I rarely followed them. All those diets ever really did was focus my mind on what I was not supposed to do. And the knock-on effect was that the more I was told I couldn't have any sugar or whatever, the more I craved it. Everything I was not meant to do became the obsession and, as for so many others, dieting never worked for me.

Motherhood and the big wake-up call

Getting pregnant was a wonderful time in my life and I genuinely enjoyed the experience. I tried not to let my weight gain become an issue because I was really excited about becoming a mum for the first time. But it was always there in the back of my mind. I think it was easier just to ignore it and carry on with the same bad eating habits I had developed over the years. Sometimes reality can be very hard to face up to.

However, having a child filled me with new responsibilities, and it was soon after Sophie's birth, when I was taking her for a short walk to the park, that I finally realised it was time to take control. That simple walk that lasted 20 minutes was a nightmare. I thought I was going to have a heart attack. The consequences of being overweight finally dawned on me. My face was purple and I was breathless. I had come out in a rash on the inside of my legs, which were swollen, and I felt exhausted. I looked at Sophie and thought, I can't do this. If Sophie grows up and sees me like this she will be embarrassed. I sat down on a bench and looked around at the other young mums. They had a pep in their step. They were laughing and running around with their children, full of life and energy. I didn't want to be a lazy mum who couldn't help her child up onto the climbing frame or chase her around the garden. And I certainly didn't want to pass on my bad eating habits to her.

That day in the park was a serious reality check. The routine that I had become trapped in had to change. I no longer wanted to wear a jumper around my waist in order to hide my spare tyre or constantly ignore my tummy hanging out over my trousers. I wanted to be in control again. In an ideal world that lightbulb moment should have been enough to make the excess pounds miraculously disappear, but unfortunately that's not real life. Making the decision to lose weight was easy. Carrying it out was much more difficult. All of my past attempts had failed and I really didn't believe in going down the road of a crash diet. I had already tried that without success. This time there really was to be no going back. This had to be a lifestyle change.

One day a woman I knew came into work looking to buy a white linen trouser suit. She was previously a big girl but that day when she walked thorugh the door I barely recognised her. She had dropped at least two dress sizes since I had last seen her. She had a glow and energy about her that was never there before. I asked her how she'd done it and she told me about a personal trainer called Dominic. She had begun to work out twice a week with him and the results were starting to pay off. I got his number a month later and called him. And so the battle to get the weight off began.

Changing my life for the better

In the early days of my new regime I remember the morning knock on the door and how I would come up with every excuse under the sun to avoid the training: I didn't sleep, Sophie wasn't well... you name it, I tried it! I think those early days were the toughest. It's the best feeling in the world to have made the decision to lose weight, but the follow-through is not as easy. After just one day of exercise I felt like giving up – the pain was unbelievable. In the beginning we did lots of walking and I remember how I had to keep stopping just so I could breathe. It took time and a lot of willpower for me to keep going. As time went on I started to take fewer breaks and, after a couple of months, that walk turned into a slow jog. Finally, after a lot of hard work and some serious detemination, that jog

Making the decision to lose weight was easy. Carrying it out was more difficult.

> *And the good news is that in ten years
> I haven't put the weight back on.*

became a sprint. The aches and pains I felt were tremendous, but the amazing thing about the pain was that I learned to love it. It was proof that what I was doing was working and I needed that to keep me motivated.

In the early months I kept a food diary and at first I was shocked by how much I was eating. I was consuming over 3,000 calories a day – more than a man should! This was an eye-opener and once I started to analyse my food I realised that much of what I was eating was not nutritious. Most of the food I was eating was laden with saturated fat and sugar, and on top of that I was still enjoying my wine or rum and coke on nights out. I was carrying on as if I had no 'stop' button. I really believe that by then food had become an addiction for me; the more I had, the more I craved.

Here's the bit that might come as a shock. It took me three years to lose 4 stone. There were a couple of times when I slipped back into my old eating habits because I got excited by my weight loss and thought it would be OK to relax a little. But it wasn't worth it, and when I felt a moment like that coming on I really focused in on the idea of this being a way of living. Losing weight is a mindset and every day is a new challenge where you are faced with making the right food choices. I had to keep reminding myself of this. It was a long journey, and it was tough, but I firmly believe that making a lifestyle change is the only way to do it. And the good news is that in ten years I haven't put the weight back on. I am still motivated by what I achieved, but the difference is I am so much more relaxed now.

Getting my confidence back

So what changed when I started to lose weight? Well, most important, my confidence began to come back. I began to feel better about myself. I re-invented my style. I now had the chance to experiment with clothes again and it was a great feeling. I no longer found myself hiding behind cardigans, tunics and scarves. I was showing off my figure and embracing all that I had achieved. I can't even begin to describe that moment when you try on clothes that you never thought would fit or suit you. It is one of those things that you just have to experience for yourself. If I could have bottled that feeling there and then I would have.

I attended a two-day motivational course with the self-help author Tony Robbins in London that started at seven in the morning and finished at midnight. At that point I realised I was high on energy. I didn't have a huge amount of food while I was there, just healthy portions. I made the decision there and then to change my life and my career. This was now about more than my weight loss. I wanted to be the very best that I could be.

I no longer found myself hiding behind cardigans, tunics and scarves. I was showing off my figure and embracing all that I had achieved.

Chapter two

Facing up
TO THE TRUTH

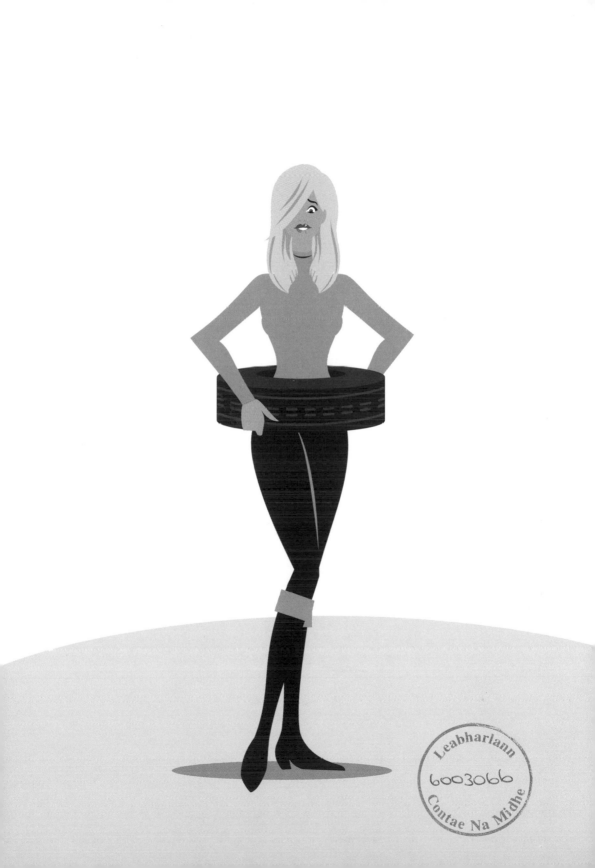

'More than ever, we as parents and a nation must do something about the growth of obesity in our children. We must do more than just talk, we must be concerned enough to act.' Lee Haney

A government report published in 2013 showed that in England most people are overweight or obese. This includes 61.3 per cent of adults and 30 per cent of children aged between two and 15. And in Australia, a report carried out in 2012 by the Council of Australian Governments showed that 63.2 per cent of Australian adults were considered overweight or obese. According to the Department of Health in Ireland, 37 per cent of adults are overweight and 24 per cent are obese.

As if those figures are not scary enough, it is estimated that 300,000 children are overweight in Ireland and that figure is rising at a rate of 10,000 per year. Ireland has the second highest obesity rates in Europe after the UK. Children who are obese are more likely to develop cardiovascular diseases such as high blood pressure and high cholesterol. They are also at a much higher risk of developing prediabetes. This occurs when your blood sugar levels are higher than they should be, but not high enough to be diagnosed with diabetes. Looking at the facts is terrifying and they are no longer something we can ignore.

My proudest achievements in life are my two children. They make me smile every single day (well, most days!) and I always cherish them. It's for that very reason that I am completely and utterly in favour of educating our young people from a very early age about health and nutrition. I think it's my duty as a mum. In light of the obesity epidemic that is raging all over the world, I think now more than ever we must take our children's health seriously.

Childhood obesity… a growing problem

How can you expect your child to learn from you if you are overweight yourself? How can you expect them to eat well if you live on junk food? We must learn to practise what we preach. So much of what young people absorb happens in the very early stages of their life. If, in those formative years, they are fed the wrong foods and develop bad eating habits, it becomes so much harder to correct the problem when they get older.

If you are in a routine that involves too much processed food, it's time to stop. Teach your children about vegetables, protein and what they need to develop strong and healthy bodies. Don't take for granted that they are being taught this in schools.

Luckily the education system in the UK and Ireland has come on in leaps and bounds. Healthy eating policies have been put in place that help to teach our children about the importance of being healthy. Most schools do not allow daily treats. In the US there are numerous campaigns to try to tackle what has become an epidemic. Groups such as Shape Up and Obesity Campaign are focusing on the changes that need to be made in order to help with the issue. In Australia they are also battling with the growing rates of childhood obesity and trying to teach children from an early age about the importance of being fit and healthy.

While these are extremely positive initiatives, I still believe it is ultimately up to the parents to take responsibility. And we can all start by making sure that our children have a good breakfast, like you, when they go out the door in the morning. Breakfast is the most important meal of their day and you have full control over it. Eating well at this time will help to boost your childen's concentration and they will be less likely to crave snacks before lunchtime. Porridge is a great way for them to start the day, and when you put some fruit like blueberries or blackberries and honey on top it's even better.

Very often parents complain that their children are fussy eaters, but this can be an excuse. If your child will only eat a limited number of foods, it's time to introduce something new. We have so many options when it comes to fruit and vegetables that you are bound to find some that they like. I always encourage my kids to try new things. If they see that you're eating it too, you're in a much stronger position to preach! Another tip that usually works is to involve them in the cooking. If they feel part of the process, they are more likely to eat the food and also they'll be open to tasting something new.

How can you expect your child to learn from you if you are overweight yourself?

Keep unhealthy snacks to a minimum. Children shouldn't have them every day and if they are you need to find a way of cutting back on this habit. Snacks should be viewed as a treat – something to enjoy at the weekend, which they look forward to, not an everyday unhealthy routine. Make a big deal of the treat. I usually tell the kids we are getting a pizza or their favourite food in advance, and then make a point of sitting down to watch a film with them. That way, the focus is not solely on what they're eating.

While you are on the way to losing weight, your children can also become part of your fitness regime. Simple things like a walk in the park or on the beach are great ways of staying active and promoting fitness. Take the stairs instead of the lift or the escalator. Walk to the shops with them rather than always jumping into the car. Make sure that they always carry a little bottle of water with them. We also tell our children, 'When you feel full, you are full.' Small changes are key to making a difference in your life and the lives of your children.

How being overweight affects your health

'Women are like tea bags. We don't know our true strength until we are in hot water!'

Eleanor Roosevelt

For so many of us women, life has its ups and downs. It might sound a bit dramatic to the men out there, but – let's be honest – it often feels like we drew the short straw. Even though I am a positive person I have to say that being a woman is sometimes tough! From a relatively young age we are faced with periods and premenstrual syndrome (PMS). Gynaecologists estimate that at least 85 per cent of women experience one or more symptoms as part of their monthly cycle. We learn to adjust to this because we have to, and eventually many of us move on to the next stage in our lives... pregnancy.

Fertility

A staggering one in six Irish and English couples who are of reproductive age will experience difficulties conceiving. According to the Fertility Society of Australia and Reuters Health in the US, that figure of one in six couples who have fertility problems is the same in their countries. While many of us are happy to bury our head in the sand in the hope that the problem will rectify itself, you can see for yourself that the figures for couples who are struggling to conceive is quite high. And, don't get me wrong, not all of the reasons for fertility problems come down to being overweight. However, it can play a part. If someone had told me that years ago, I'd like to think I would have taken their advice on board. Before I continue I want to reinforce that what I am advocating here is a lifestyle change. I'm trying to convince you that being overweight is not good for you and, if you are trying for a baby, it's more important than ever that you make a change.

Recent research carried out by the Nurses' Health Study shows that obesity does have reproductive consequences. In fact, it suggests that 25 per cent of ovulatory infertility in the US may be attributable to obesity. Being overweight has so many consequences – it affects our menstrual cycle, disrupts ovulation and, in severe cases, stops it altogether. Being overweight means you are carrying excess fat tissue, which can lead to you producing too much oestrogen. And excess oestrogen can cause hormonal imbalances that can affect ovulation. The reality is that by losing weight you are more likely to regulate your hormones, which means that the chances of conception will be higher. You will also be in a better position to experience a healthy pregnancy.

Looking after myself is the one thing I learnt to do when I was trying for my second child, Dalton. I knew what I should and shouldn't be eating – and so should you. A recent study has shown that the type of carbohydrates you eat can have an effect on fertility. As you may already know, there are fast and slow carbs.

Being overweight has so many consequences – it affects our menstrual cycle, disrupts ovulation and, in severe cases, stops it altogether.

The fast ones are broken down or digested easily and give you quick bursts of energy. They produce insulin and when this insulin level is too high it interferes with the hormonal balance that you need for fertility. Fast carbs are white bread, white pasta, cakes and chips. Basically they are all the wrong foods that I lived on before I saw sense! So the good news is that you can still eat carbs, but they need to be the slow type. These release energy slowly and keep your blood sugar at a stable level. Slow carbs include wholegrains, vegetables, chicken, beans, egg whites and many more.

If you are currently in the process of trying to conceive, it's always a good idea to consult your GP before starting a weight-loss programme. Always consult your doctor, too, if you are already pregnant, since sudden weight loss can be dangerous for your baby.

My pregnancy and pre-eclampsia

If I have yet to convince you that weight loss is vital when trying to conceive, please try to take this next piece of information on board. Being overweight can increase your risk of diabetes, pre-eclampsia and also your chance of needing to have a caesarean section. I'm going to tell you a little about my own experience as unfortunately I did get pre-eclampsia with Sophie. Even thinking about that now is quite upsetting because I know that it was something I could have prevented.

I found being pregnant with Sophie very tough because I was overweight. I certainly didn't feel like a poster mum-to-be! I was incredibly uncomfortable and I can vividly remember the feeling of my thighs rubbling together and the rash I got on my legs. On the second last visit to my gynaecologist he broke the news to me that I had pre-eclampsia. Deep down I had known something was wrong, but I didn't want to let myself believe it. This was my first pregnancy, Paul and I were becoming parents for the first time, and I wanted everything to be just right.

I'm hoping that this story resonates with some of you so that you never end up in the situation I was in. Being overweight at that time had a negative effect on my pregnancy and it's something I could have prevented, which is why I made sure it did not happen again when I became pregnant for the second time. All the things you need to do to look after yourself are common sense. And, yes, it comes down to you being a healthy weight and eating sensibly, so please don't ignore this important advice. I know only too well that feeling of being a mum for the first time. Of course, you will have worries and insecurities. You're not normal if you don't. But give yourself the best possible chance you can and, if you need to make changes, start today before it's too late.

The menopause

The last card we are dealt as women is the dreaded menopause. For most women this usually happens between the ages of 48 and 55 and the symptoms are different for all of us. The menopause is defined as the point in a woman's life when her menstruation finally stops. Now here is the bit that once again you might not like me saying – your weight will have an effect on your menopause. So many changes occur in your life around this time that being overweight will only contribute to them. You are not superhuman, so don't try to solve everything immediately. You're going to experience erratic periods, night sweats and hot flushes caused by changes in your hormones as well as feeling more emotional than usual. You'll experience fluctuating moods and find that you're possibly not as tolerant as you were before. The menopause may also have an impact on your libido. These are major things for a woman to go through, so it's just as well they don't all happen at once. Most women experience premenopausal symptoms like those above years before the menopause comes on fully.

The other major change that women often experience around this time is weight gain. So it stands to reason that if you are already overweight, the issue will be increased. The menopause brings with it a decrease in your oestrogen levels and your metabolism starts to slow down, which means that it will become harder for you to lose weight. More than ever at this time, exercise needs to be a part of your lifestyle. It's not enough just to watch what you eat, because what you will notice is that most of the excess weight you are carrying is in one place – and that is around the tummy area. A good mix of exercise would be some aerobic activity, such as swimming, walking or cycling, as well as strength training,

The last card we are dealt as women is the dreaded menopause.

By the time you reach this stage in your life it's likely that your metabolism will have slowed down by more than 20 per cent.

such as using weights or gym equipment. Join a class or begin a workout regime at home. Just get active.

By the time you reach this stage in your life it's likely that your metabolism will have slowed down by more than 20 per cent. I don't know about you, but that scares me! I think sometimes we believe we are invincible, but there is no denying the ageing process and all that goes with it. Therefore you have to take your diet into consideration. Try to practise sensible portion control and get a good mix of protein and fibre. You'll find these foods fill you up more, so you'll be less inclined to reach for the fat and sugar. Also be aware of the time of day you are eating. This really comes into play during menopause and many women find themselves snacking throughout the day and into the night. Eating well earlier in the day will put a stop to this. I would recommend not eating after 7pm unless it's fruit or nuts.

Managing stress needs to be top of your list, especially if you feel your levels rising. There is definitely a link between food and mood, and if you are struggling you will be more inclined to reach for the wrong types. I always think that coping with stress means getting to know yourself a bit better. Try to recognise the signs when you feel under pressure. If you learn to anticipate them, you will be in a better position to control them. Also make sure that you try to get a good night's sleep every night. I'm a big believer in this one, and it's something I rarely falter on.

I'm not saying that all of these tips will help you sail through menopause with a flat belly and a spring in your step, but I hope they will encourage you to approach this stage in your life with gusto. Talk to your friends, be honest about what you are going through and feel the relief of knowing that you're not alone. Above all, don't get to this stage and try to deal with your weight on top of all the other symptoms you have to contend with.

Middle-age spread

We have all heard of the middle-age spread and it's not a myth! Many men and women sail through their twenties and thirties without problems developing around the midriff. But as we reach our late thirties the cracks can begin to appear. In fact, because of environmental and dietary factors, it seems to be happening at an even younger age for some. Women who have never carried weight are suddenly landed with this bulge around their middle.

What happens naturally as we grow older is that our metabolism starts to slow down. We don't require as many calories and yet we often find we eat the same amount, if not more. At the same time, many of us may not be quite as active as we were when we were younger.

Weight around our tummy is both harder to shift and poses certain health risks due to the fact that it collects around our abdominal organs. So it's important to understand that carrying weight around the tummy is not only unattractive, but also it could be damaging to your health – for example, it is associated with a number of cardiovascular problems such as heart disease and stroke, as well as type 2 diabetes. The positive news is that it is possible both to reverse and prevent middle-age spread through a mixture of healthy eating and exercise.

Eating well goes without saying. However, the bottom line is that now that your metabolism has slowed down you simply cannot consume more energy than you are likely to burn off, otherwise the effects will show! Now, more than ever, you really need to learn the art of eating well and recognising when you are full. Fibre, vegetables and fruit are what you need to stock up on to prevent further weight gain around the tummy area. You will also see results if you eliminate fatty, processed and sugary foods. In particular, if you cut out white bread completely.

We have all heard of the middle-age spread and it's not a myth!

You have to exercise as well. Don't think that just because you have been lucky up until now you will continue to be! Exercise can be especially hard for women who have never included it as part of their routine. However, once you get started and see the results it will be easier to keep going. Stay active in all aspects of your life and get as much aerobic exercise as you can. You need to be working out at least three or four times a week. Even if you hate it at first, persevere because it is worth it. You will find that you feel much healthier and better in yourself. You will probably begin to sleep better as well. This is really important because stress and lack of rest do not help with the middle-age spread. I may not enjoy the exercise, but I love the results. They are what give me the strength to keep going!

When it comes to alcohol, women often find that they enjoy their wine that bit more as they get older! The bad news is that it can be disastrous for our midriff. They don't call it a 'beer belly' for no reason! Drinking alcohol causes fatty deposits around our middle and, for many, also excess fat known as a double chin. Eliminating alcohol from our diet is one way to control our weight gain, but that is quite a drastic measure. A more realistic approach is to become aware of the effects alcohol can have on your weight. Simple steps such as choosing a drink that is low in calories (see page 72) or sticking to soda water with spirits is one thing you can do to help. I usually alternate between wine and vodka on different days, adding sparkling water and fresh lime juice when you have a mixer because these contain fewer calories. I also frequently add soda water or sparkling water to wine to turn it into a spritzer. One of the worst things that you can do is to drink on an empty stomach. And don't drink too late at night as it means there is less time to burn off the calories. If I drink a glass of water after every glass of wine I drink less. It is possible to take charge of middle-age spread – just start acting right now!

Keep active and get as much aerobic exercise as you can.

You have to exercise as well. Don't think that just because you have been lucky up until now you will continue to be! Exercise can be especially hard for women who have never included it as part of their routine. However, once you get started and see the results it will be easier to keep going.

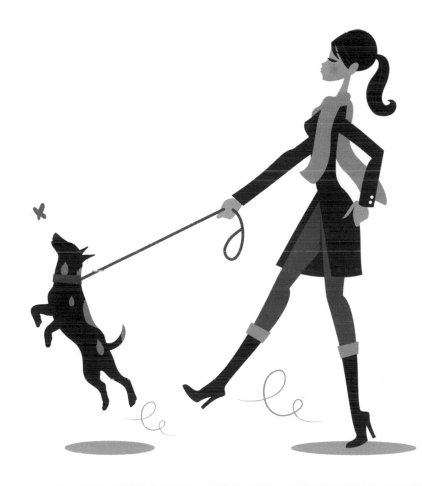

Chapter three

Start being
HONEST WITH YOURSELF

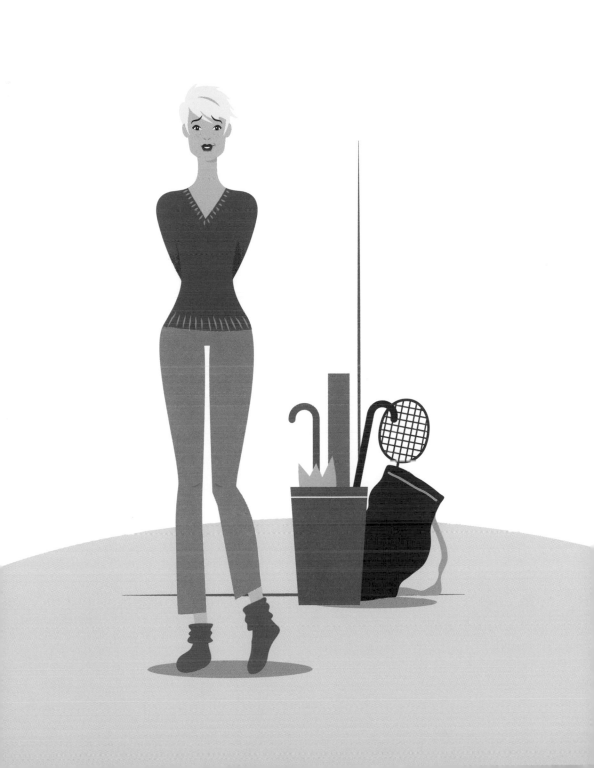

You don't suddenly wake up one morning and discover that you're overweight.

You only have yourself to blame for being overweight. This may sound a bit harsh when you read it for the first time, but deep down you know that it's true. Unless you have been diagnosed with a medical condition that has caused you to gain weight, you have to take responsibility for your situation. I've said before that I was probably in denial for a long time before I was ready to face up to the fact that my weight had spiralled out of control. I know that back then food was my comfort; however, admitting it had become a problem was one of the toughest things I've ever had to do. Saying that, there was only one person who could fix the situation and that was me. I never blamed anyone else for the size I was. I got there all by myself! It didn't happen overnight. The weight crept up slowly – something that many of you can probably empathise with. You don't suddenly wake up one morning and discover that you're overweight. You may not want to hear it but you are the only person who can take control. It's easy to blame our genes or our partner's eating habits or our unfortunate metabolism, but the bottom line is that, if you want to lose weight you have to set yourself that goal and make it a reality.

If you are looking for a miracle, you'll be left waiting! I spent years hoping that my weight problems would just disappear. I'd talk about dieting, but never actually got round to doing anything about it. I'd buy the running gear and never take it out of the bags. I'm sure this may sound familiar to many of you. Only when I made the decision to do something about it did the change come. It is possible, but you have to want to do it. Stop feeling sorry for yourself and comparing your situation to that of others. There is no secret fix or magic diet pill that will miraculously solve your problems. They simply don't exist. Of course, you can continue to be lured into the latest craze, for as long you like, but the truth is that you will only lose weight by eating well and exercising. It's the cheapest and healthiest option. What you need is determination and discipline. Nothing else will work.

Can you really be fat and happy?

Sometimes you hear people refer to a woman who is overweight as having a bubbly personality. I suppose this has become a term that rightly or wrongly we now associate with larger ladies. But does the word 'bubbly' really describe how some of these women feel? Are they good at putting on an act or are they genuinely happy? It's a tough one because only they can answer that question. Maybe you genuinely are the happiest person in the world, but having walked in those shoes, so to speak, I find it hard to believe that being overweight actually does make all women completely content.

My memories of the years when I piled on the pounds are definitely filled with mixed emotions. Certain things in my life did seem perfect, but deep down I did feel like I was carrying a burden when it came to my size. It was only when I made the decision to take control of my weight that I could see things clearly. Being bigger did indeed make me feel unhappy, but I found that out only when I began to lose weight and grow in confidence. Once the weight was off, I loved the feeling of being content with everything and knowing I was giving myself the best chance possible of living life to the full. It had a massive impact on the way I viewed things and, in many ways, it was like a new way of feeling.

Looking back, my bubbly personality probably masked my weight issue. It became my 'front' when I met people. It's much easier to tell yourself that you're happy being the size you are, rather than admitting to yourself that your weight might be an issue. As I've said before, I found ways to hide behind what I wore. But that can be so draining, and I think for some it can take its toll. Behind closed doors the reality of being overweight can have a huge impact on your confidence and self-esteem. This is often when people find comfort in food, which is probably the worst thing they can do. I think that if you are one of those people who have learned how to put on a good show for others, you should never use that as a safety net to stay the way you are. It could become a habit and

There is no secret fix or magic diet pill that will miraculously solve your problems.

then you'll end up trying to convince yourself that being overweight makes you happy. You owe it to yourself to be truly happy and to live the best possible life that you can.

It may not be intentional, but sometimes those closest to us can be the worst supporters of change because they are used to us being a certain way. They may not fully understand our motives for wanting to lose weight in the first place. If this is the case in your relationship, remind yourself that this decision is all about doing *what is right for you*. If you're not sure how you feel, ask yourself the following questions:

1. **Do you like how you look?**
2. **Does your weight make you feel good about yourself?**
3. **Are you happy being fat?**

I suppose the last question is the most important one of all. Are you happy being fat? If the answer is 'no', there has never been a better time to change your life. Don't put it off until tomorrow. Grab the opportunity with both hands and make the decision to improve your situation now.

Feeling insecure

If you feel insecure in yourself on a daily basis, you are not alone. A survey carried out in the United States showed that 80 per cent of obese people who were questioned believed the following: that others perceive them to be physically unattractive, that others comment on their weight, that they are uncomfortable about being seen in public, and so on. I'd say, having been in that position, that this survey is pretty accurate.

Through my work I meet women all the time who talk to me, confide in me and look for answers about what suits their body shape and size. Often they approach me to talk about style, but very often they ask for advice on how they can cover up parts of their body they don't like. Now, as I've said before, covering up your bad bits is fine – we all do it. However, when it gets to a point where we are hiding from ourselves, we need to address the problem. Of course, it's fine to cover up short term until you are in a position where you no longer have to. But I don't want you to spend countless years trying to cover up everything, constantly worried about who is looking at you and what they are thinking. I did that for six years and it wasn't a nice feeling. I want you to get to a point in your life where you can stand proud, be the weight you want to be and be unaffected by what others think. Start by working on your good areas and then learn to hide the bad. We all have different goals – it's up to you to plan yours now.

How being overweight can affect relationships

I mentioned earlier that Paul doesn't remember me when I was overweight. Thank God, is all I can say! He loved me just the same as when he first met me and for that I feel extremely lucky. When he looked at me he saw 'Lisa' and not 'overweight Lisa', which was who I stared at in the mirror. My insecurities did not come from anything he said or did. I simply built them up in my head, allowing the weight to win constantly. As much as Paul loved me, it wasn't up to him to solve my insecurities. If you want to make a positive change in your life, do it because you want to become healthier and happier. I always say to brides-to-be, 'Your fiancé loves you now for who you are and has committed to you for a life together. Don't lose weight to fit into your wedding dress.'

If you are in a relationship

If you are seeing someone and you have started on this weight-loss journey, try not to let it dominate the time you spend together. Don't discuss it at every waking moment or become obsessed by it. Of course, you are allowed to talk about it – just do it in moderation. Remember:

- Your relationship must come first.
- Don't let your weight battle affect your love life.
- Try to view what you're doing as positive.
- When low self-esteem or negative thoughts begin to creep in, have a good old talking to yourself and realise that your thoughts can have a positive effect.

I want you to get to a point in your life where you can stand proud, be the weight you want to be and be unaffected by what others think.

If you are happy being single

If you are single and happy that way, good for you – as long as you are not single and wallowing in the fact that you're overweight and without a partner.

- Remind yourself that being overweight does not stop you from meeting new people or forming new friendships or relationships. However, your negativity does have the power to do that.
- Be someone who grabs opportunities in life and takes chances in order to push yourself. I like to be challenged and try to do this quite a lot. It's what keeps me motivated!
- Don't be afraid to put yourself out there and be sociable. Join a group or some kind of club that forces you into a new situation. It's good for your head, good for your self-esteem and good for your emotional wellbeing.

Relationships with friends and family

Other relationships that can be affected by your weight are those with family and friends. Some will be supportive and others won't. Focus on the people who are encouraging you to lose weight and whose opinion you value. Years ago, a friend of mine whom I hadn't seen in a while said to me, 'Oh my god, you've put on weight'. I was completely taken aback. Just what every girl wants to hear when they are struggling with excess bulge! Of course what he said hurt, but he didn't mean to upset me. It was a truthful and genuine observation. I had put on weight. My reaction could have been to take what he said to heart and not to talk to him again, but then I'd have lost a good friend and to me it wasn't worth it. Thank you, Louis Walsh, a true pal and always honest!

Work relationships

For some of you, work will be a part of your life that may increase your insecurities. It's a place where you have to face people every day and that's not easy when your weight is always dominating your thoughts. Without being harsh, try to use this as further motivation for change. If you let your insecurities consume you, whatever you are doing in the work environment is going to suffer. No one wants to be in a position where their weight impacts their career. Go in every day with a smile on your face, safe in the knowledge that you are going to lose the weight. It will result in you feeling better about yourself and the chances of you excelling in work will be higher because you will have developed a new-found confidence.

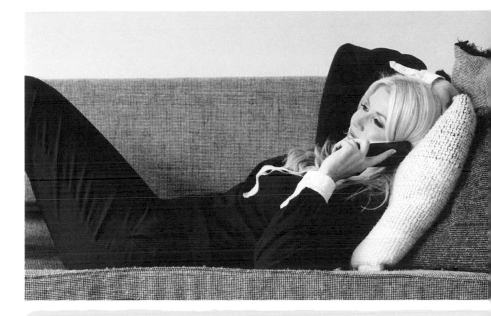

Choosing your support network wisely

Once I decided to lose weight I did pretty much go it alone. I didn't shout it from the rooftops, because I didn't want the pressure of people watching me and waiting for the weight to fall off. Of course I told my husband Paul, my mum and my close friends, but that was where I left it. You might want to open up to a few people and share your plan. The decision is entirely up to you and only you know what will work best for you. You will find this tough, but if you have some support it will definitely make it easier. It can be useful to have a shoulder to cry on, encouragement to keep you going and also someone to tell you to step away from the biscuit tin! If there is somebody else who is ready to embark on this journey with you, even better. Your family and friends are the people who know you inside out, who love you no matter what and who hopefully realise just how important this is to you. Laugh with them, cry with them and, if you need to, lean on them.

Chapter four

Changing
YOUR LIFE AROUND

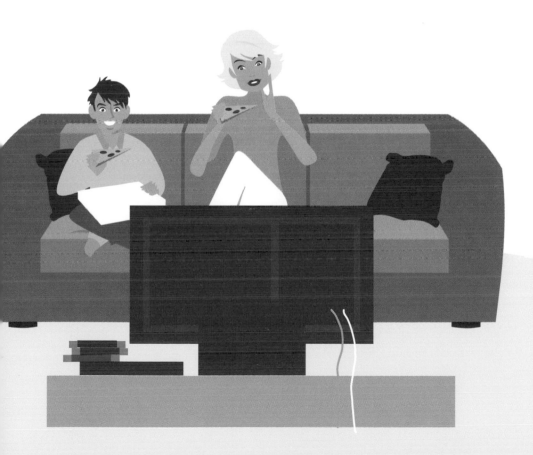

Stop talking about it and make it happen.

It's your body, your responsibility. Sometimes in life we need a wake-up call. I told you about my defining moment being when I looked at my beautiful baby daughter Sophie and realised how losing weight had to become my priority. I loved her too much and wanted to be the very best version of me that I possibly could. Often I ask myself why it took me up to that point to become aware of what was probably obvious to those around me. I discovered that it was important for me to ake the decision for myself because that was what I wanted, because I had arrived at a point where it was the right time for me and nobody else. It's probably the reason you are reading this book. The reality is that everyone has to find something that strikes a chord with them.

Try to find the motivation from somewhere to get you started. Focus on the reason why you want to lose weight. Will your life improve if you do? Will you feel better in yourself? Will you be healthier? Will you look better? The answer to these questions is 'yes', in case you're not sure. I should know! But you have to arrive at that place all by yourself. There is no secret to being fit and healthy. You just have to get out and do it. Stop talking about it and make it happen. There is no better time than now. Start slowly, but do get started. The more slowly you lose the weight the more slowly you will put it back on. But if you stay positive and focused you should keep it off for good.

The dreaded 'D' word

The easiest thing in the world can be to hide away from a problem. We say to ourselves 'I'll deal with it tomorrow' or 'I'm tired' because we don't want to face up to things. And who could blame us? Diets can be a form of torture. According to Cover Me, a Canadian insurance company, statistics show that '85 per cent of people will lose weight on a diet, but only 15 per cent will keep it off after two years'. Some people gain back even more weight than they originally lost. A recent survey carried out by a home delivery diet brand, Diet Chef, found that the average woman spends nearly two decades of her life on a diet. Well, I would argue more!

How many times on a Monday morning have you heard the words, 'The diet starts today'? How many women start a diet every year on 1 January? Research shows that barely two weeks later, 42 per cent have quit. Talking about the diet becomes more of a focus than the act itself. And when we are actually on the diet we tell ourselves all sorts of crazy things: it doesn't count as a dessert if it contains fruit; it's fine to eat a burger and chips if I eat the side salad as well; chocolate is made with milk therefore it has some goodness; diet cola is healthy because it says 'diet' on the front... The list is endless and eventually you start to convince yourself that these things are true.

Five step plan for change

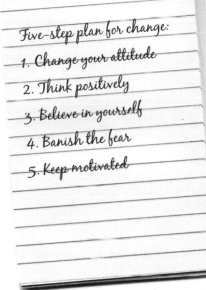

Five-step plan for change:
1. Change your attitude
2. Think positively
3. Believe in yourself
4. Banish the fear
5. Keep motivated

1 Change your attitude

Do not feel bad if you have tried a million diets and you still weigh the same, if not more than before you started. Diets are often why people fail. In many cases they are unachievable and they don't focus on a realistic lifestyle change. Don't get me started on the fact that many involve the most impossible rules. What I want you to do is to try to forget what happened to your weight in the past. You are starting afresh. This is all about developing the right attitude towards your health and not about dropping a dress size in a week – first and foremost, that is unhealthy and, second, it plays havoc with your emotions. You diet, lose those pounds, wear the amazing dress without bursting out and then a week later the diet is finished and you're back to square one. It's like giving a child an amazing toy for Christmas and then taking it back after a day! This has to be about an attitude that lasts, and not a quick fix.

Remember that this is your journey. We have a terrible habit of looking around and comparing ourselves to others. We want their toned legs, flat tummy, silky hair, gorgeous eyes, etc. You need to make a conscious decision right now to stop doing this, as it can be destructive. By all means admire and compliment others, but not to the point where you wish you looked like them. You are you! You have to learn to be complete with you. If you accept yourself for who you are, you will feel better about yourself.

② Think positively

Start by focusing on all the positive things in your life. I am a naturally 'glass half full' kind of person. Don't get me wrong, I have my moments when I might think the world is against me, but for the most part I look on the bright side. The question is how do you take control and ensure your positive thoughts are the dominant ones when it feels like the odds are stacked against you? You have to change your way of thinking and allow the good thoughts to be in charge. You have to decide what you want and then do what it takes to make that happen.

Here is the first thing I will ask of you. Can you write down ten good things that you have in your life? Depending on your mood, this may or may not be a difficult task! Take your time and really allow yourself to think about what makes you happy. Don't tell me you can't think of anything because I know you can! My list would include family, friends, work, meeting new people, holidays with the kids, music, sunny days, dates with my husband, nights on the couch in my pyjamas and laughing with friends.

The reason it's good to make a list is that it allows you to see the bigger picture in relation to your weight loss. Being overweight and feeling discontented is something that has the power to dominate everything. We find ourselves in a place where we are unable to think about anything else, where we feel everyone is talking about us and our confidence hits rock bottom. The harsh reality is that most people don't care about how you feel. That's not me being cruel; it's just the way of the world. People have their own problems; they are busy going about their daily life and whether or not you have gained 5lb is irrelevant to them.

Stop worrying about what other people may or may not think of you. It is a serious waste of time and energy, not to mention having a negative effect on you. This process starts with you. It means switching off all those paranoid thoughts and starting to appreciate the good things. I can almost guarantee that if you took the weight out of the equation you would be able to do this without much difficulty. But right now it is a stumbling block, so you have to find a way of not letting it define who you are. It's only part of you and you have so much more going for you.

Once you have made your list, I want you to read it back to yourself. Read it out loud, hear the words and believe them. These are the wonderful things that you have in your life. They are the things to be thankful for. As we continue with this process I am going to ask you to recite this list every morning and every evening. I know it may seem a little forced, and you may not feel like doing it every day, but it is certainly a way of encouraging a positive state of mind. All I can say is give it a try. It will not work overnight and you have to persevere. But hopefully after a while your perspective will change and your thoughts won't always be clouded by your weight.

Our ability to stay positive has a lot to do with the people we surround ourselves with, so the lesson here is choose your friends carefully! If you want to become a positive person, you have to make sure you spend time with other people who have a similar outlook. They are people who rarely use the word 'can't' and who will never drain you of energy. They have a passion and a zest for everything and they are worth knowing!

3 Believe in yourself

Very often the people who are successful in life are not the most skilled or talented. They are the people who believe in themselves. They believe that anything is possible and that attitude puts them ahead of the rest. That belief is a choice that every single one of us is free to make. The sooner you start to believe in yourself, the sooner things in your life will start to change.

When I developed that belief in myself again I got my confidence back. I realised how years ago it was my insecurity that caused me to have an issue around my education. I have learned now that just because I didn't go to college,

Stop worrying about what other people may or may not think of you. It is a serious waste of time and energy, not to mention having a negative effect on you.

it doesn't mean that I am not a capable person. I let go of that hang-up and used it to do something positive. I have recently completed a course in cognitive behaviour therapy and it was a great experience.

Don't push aside the things that you want to achieve just because you are not completely happy with how you look. Don't let your weight stop you from achieving things right now. You have made the step towards a new you, so there is no better time to believe in yourself. Be it in your work, home or love life, you have the ability to do anything you want. Begin working on it now.

Banish the fear

Our fear of failing is often responsible for us not even trying. You have to learn to see past the fear and seize the day. Living a full life and achieving our goals is what we should all be doing. Of course you have insecurities – who doesn't? But fearing something that might not even happen is a real waste of time. It won't change anything. All it does is play with your mind and prevent you from being happy. The thing to realise is that while fear is natural, it should never hold you back from fulfilling your dreams.

I have learned over time that fear can be turned into something positive. I don't let it stop me trying new things. Instead, I use fear as a trigger to challenge myself further because I like the feeling it gives me. I genuinely believe that it is my determination to overcome my fears that has made me a stronger person.

Keep motivated

The question I am asked most often is: 'How did you get motivated?' Of course, the motivation for reading this will be different for each and every one of you. However, my biggest motivation was my children. When you become a parent for the first time, your priorities naturally change and you come to realise that, above all, your responsibility is to look after your own. My goal was quite simple: to become fit and healthy. For me, losing weight wasn't an option; it was a necessity.

When setting goals, the most important thing is to make sure they are realistic.

When setting goals, the most important thing is to make sure they are realistic. Take one day at a time and write down tomorrow's list of goals the night before. Look at your list the following morning and try to keep your objectives fresh in your head throughout the day. Sometimes I jot down a reminder about healthy eating, so my list will include a note to bring my lunch with me to avoid making the wrong choices when I'm on the go, or I'll make a note to call a friend whom I haven't spoken to for a while. Try not to focus all of your energy on losing weight; in order to stay positive, it's important to shift your attention away from your weight loss to other areas of your life as well.

Stay focused on your goal at all times. I have heard many times about putting a 'fat photo' of yourself on the fridge to encourage you to keep going. Well, I suggest you do the opposite and choose a picture of yourself that you love – one that reminds you of a happy time when you were comfortable with your body and life was good. The incentive is to get back to that time when you felt great about yourself. I did this when I was starting out; I placed my photo on the fridge as a constant reminder of why I was doing what I was doing; I found that it put a more positive slant on things. If you have never felt comfortable with your body, and you don't have a picture, the power of visualisation can be very effective. Imagine how you want to look and let that be your goal.

My tips for staying motivated

Apart from writing out your daily goals the night before, what else can you do to kickstart this new motivated you? Here are my top tips:

 Choose a mantra: Come up with a phrase that best describes the journey you are embarking on – for example, 'I look great and I am on the way to a healthier me,' or 'I'm feeling positive and I am achieving my goals one day at a time.' Repeat your mantra as many times as you can during the day. Say it out loud, if possible, but constantly have it in your head so that it becomes your way of thinking. Positive affirmations have the power to challenge any negative thoughts or self-doubt that might be creeping in. They also have the power to keep you focused on your inner goals. Mine is 'I like me and I'm a good person.' If you have tried using affirmations before and it hasn't worked, I would encourage you to give it another go. This time you are making a lifestyle choice and there are so many things that you have the power to change. You have to be consistent, though. It will only work if you practise it on a daily basis.

Remember to treat yourself: As the old saying goes, 'A little of what you fancy won't do you any harm.' If you deprive yourself of what you love, I can assure you that your cravings will be ten times worse! So learn how to limit what you eat. I do this by eating healthily during the week and allowing myself some time out at the weekend: it's basically, 'bye bye Healthy, hello Friday!' Of course, I don't always go mad, but it's about a mindset: I'm not depriving myself completely, it's just that if I want a treat I have to wait until the weekend. The best advice I can give you here is to enjoy that time as best you can. Don't feel guilty – it defeats the purpose.

Don't be too hard on yourself: It's easy to have a bad day, or even bad moments, but don't dwell on them. Instead, learn to move on and remember all the good things you are doing to change your lifestyle. Along the way, it's important to keep patting yourself on the back for what you are achieving. The best feeling in the world is when someone comments on your weight loss. Take the compliment and recognise what you have done so far. That is often motivation enough to keep you going on your journey. Remember: you will have setbacks. The most important thing is to get back up and start again immediately.

Create a wish list of other things you want in life: One of the best things I do is create wish lists. I try to do it every year and include things I want to achieve in my career or personal life. I have to say it has really worked for me and I've found myself being able to tick off so many things. It's empowering, a great way of getting focused, and it also takes the attention away from your weight loss. You find yourself thinking of all the things you would like to do or achieve and this creates a positive energy. Take that a step further and imagine the feeling of actually crossing off things on your wish list. Believe they are possible and they will happen to you.

Find a theme tune: Pick one song that makes you want to smile, dance or jump around the room. Identify this as your theme tune and listen to it every time you need a pick-me-up. My theme tune is 'Respect', sung by Aretha Franklin. It's the song that gets me in the mood to face the day and it reminds me of the important things in life – the need to respect myself, the people I care about and my body. Choose what works for you – music can be very powerful so use it.

6 **Laugh loud and often:** The other piece of motivational advice I want to give you is to take life a little less seriously. I'm not underestimating what you're going through or dealing with; I just want you to do your best to enjoy life. It costs nothing to laugh, so you should do it more often. Surely you know somebody who can always be relied on for a good belly laugh – now is the time to take advantage. Laughter is such a good medicine and, while you are on the road to a better you, enjoying yourself will make it so much easier. If you don't believe me, listen to the legend. As the great Charlie Chaplin said, 'A day without laughter is a day wasted.'

Not all of my tips will work for you, but In time you will find the ones that suit you best. In many ways it's a journey of self-discovery and you have to stick with it, particularly during the moments when you feel like giving up.

Ignore the pressure to be slim

For some women the pressure to remain slim and seemingly perfect to the outside world just isn't an issue. They might not be perfect, as there is no such thing, but they are not affected by what other people think of them. Isn't that a great way to be? But for many of us living in today's vanity-driven world, even glimpsing a gossip magazine in our local shop could trigger

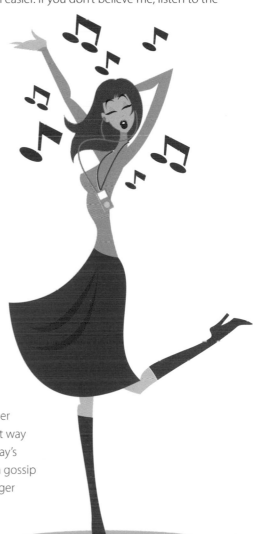

How does she stay so thin? Will I ever be that glamorous?

emotions of self-doubt and anxiety. Why don't I look like that? How does she stay so thin? Will I ever be that glamorous? Comparing ourselves to celebrities will never make us feel better, but, let's be honest, it's hard to avoid the comparison when it stares at you in the face every day. If we're not being bombarded with the latest celebrity weight-loss story, it's a supermodel who has given birth and two months later is flaunting her completely flat stomach. Then, on the flip side, we have magazines that print pictures of famous people in their bikinis who have gained weight. It seems so cruel to do this, and yet it gives some women hope that celebrities are real, just like us, and they too can pile on the pounds. Of course, our happiness shouldn't rely solely on how we look, but for most people it does matter.

When you are overweight it's easy to feel that people are talking about you or commenting on how you look. Paranoia sets in because underneath you yourself are not comfortable in your own skin. That's why some of us spend time covering up – we don't want to reveal what's underneath. I remember one of my really good friends asking me what I got for my 30th birthday. I showed her the fabulous shoes I was wearing that night and said they were a present from my husband. At the time, I thought they were amazing. Bling wasn't the word. They were literally bling-tastic and very Shirley Bassey! But, looking back, once again I see that the shoes were a symbol of what I was actually hiding. They were there to distract attention from my weight and in my head it made perfect sense. My friend wanted to know why I hadn't bought a new dress instead of shoes. I had one dress that I felt comfortable in and wore it to most occasions. My friend looked at me quite seriously and said, 'It's a shame – you're so pretty! You should try to lose weight'. I might not have felt like a size 18, but everyone around me could see it. I put a smile on my face, blew out the candles and cut myself an extremely big slice of cake. That was a moment when I can honestly say I felt the pressure; however, it didn't stop me from eating. What I'm trying to share with you is that pressure from friends, family or the media won't spur you to make a change. The desire has to come solely from you and your goals need to be clear.

So how do you avoid the pressure and figure out what makes you happy? Start by putting things into perspective, being realistic and finding a way to be confident in your own skin. Every change you make should be for you alone and nobody else – otherwise it just won't work.

- **Remember celebrities rarely have real lives:** For starters, a team of stylists, make-up artists and hair experts surround them daily. Some of them don't step outside the front door until they have been coiffed and preened within an inch of their life. How can we mere mortals live up to this and why would we even try? Yes, for the most part, celebrities appear to be super-slim and equally super-fit. But the truth is they probably work incredibly hard to achieve their figure. It's not as if the whole celebrity population is naturally a size 8! For some reason, the media feel the need to portray these women as extraordinary and in doing so put enormous pressure on real women. We should all be aware that in many cases these women have not only been styled and beautified, but also they have been airbrushed – so the pictures that you stare at in magazines have been altered. They may also have chefs and personal fitness trainers. The celebrity influence is worrying, but we have to learn not to let it win. Be inspired by celebrities who fly the flag for real women and try not to succumb to what is perceived to be beautiful by the media. Kate Winslet once said, 'I'd rather be known as curvy Kate than some skinny stick'. I have to say, I admire her attitude and her honesty.

- **Don't obsess about calorie content:** Another pressure that has recently begun to surface is restaurants displaying the calorie content of their food. Yes, it's essential that information about allergies is displayed, but I really feel providing calorie counts is a gimmick that sucks women into believing they are getting a diet or low-fat meal. Don't forget you are clever enough to know what is healthy and what isn't. If you want to choose the best option, you can. This is just another example of the constant pressure we are under to think about our weight. Once again, the pressure to lose weight is being forced on us rather than it coming from within.

- **Don't compare yourself to others:** When you're feeling vulnerable, it's all too easy to compare yourself with others. We all know the result – we end up feeling even more inadequate about how we look. From now on, I urge you to get out of the habit of not feeling good enough. Learn to love what's on the inside and start to believe in yourself and what you can achieve. Only when you learn to feel comfortable in your own skin, will you truly be happy – and that is a feeling that no one else can take away.

Exercise – where to start?

'Ability is what you're capable of doing. Motivation determines what you do. Attitude determines how well you do it.' Lou Holtz

Less talking… more action!

If you're not a naturally sporty or active person, do not despair. There is some kind of exercise out there that will suit you and, furthermore, you might shock yourself by actually enjoying it. The truth is that if you are really determined to lose weight, diet changes alone will not be enough. The two principles of diet and exercise go hand in hand. Exercise is a topic that often freaks women out. Where will I find the time? It's never worked for me before. How do I start again? Maybe you have tried, on so many occasions, to get yourself into a routine and for whatever reason it hasn't worked. The intention is always good, but the reality is somewhat different. All is not lost, though, and it is possible for you to give this another shot. Building exercise into your daily routine should become a habit like everything else you're doing. Here are my top tips for getting started:

1 **Choose an exercise that you feel will work for you and set yourself realistic goals.** The gym is a good option if you want somebody to set you up on a plan that is tailored to suit your needs. Aerobic walking and running are great ways to get fit without your bank balance being affected! Swimming, cycling, yoga, spinning, pilates, dancing, aerobics… there are so many options for you to choose from. You might have to try a few before you find what's best for you. The most important thing is to get active and increase your heart rate. Over time, this will make you fitter and your heart will become stronger.

2 **If you are taking this seriously, you should be working out for at least half an hour, three to four times a week.** Your aim should always be to increase your heart rate and get your muscles moving. All you need is a pair of good-quality trainers and a little bit of determination! Choose a pair that is suitable for the exercise you plan to do.

3 **Write down what you are setting out to achieve.** Post it on the fridge or on a mirror – just make sure it's somewhere that will provide you with a constant reminder of what you need to do. Use your diary or phone to mark in exactly when and where you are doing the chosen exercise. This means that you can't say you didn't have time or you forgot. Planning is everything. Seeing these plans written in black and white makes them real. You need to focus on following them through, taking it one day at a time.

4 **Keep a diary of what you achieve each time you exercise.** For example, if you are running, keep track of your time and distance each time you go out. Keep pushing for your personal best. It's a good way of measuring your progress and will also give you the motivation to continue. If you miss a day, do not be tempted to quit altogether. Use it as an opportunity to try harder and make up for lost ground the next time you work out.

5 **Enjoy the feeling.** Yes, you will ache a little for the first few weeks as your body adjusts to the foreign feeling of exercise! However, rest assured that this is perfectly normal. You are using muscles that haven't had a day out in a very long time, but soon it will get easier. I remember all too well thinking I couldn't physically keep going, but I persevered. Your body is amazing and it will adjust to the changes. Be patient and give it time to get used to what you are doing. View the aches and pains as a sign that you are doing something right. Your hard work is worth it!

6 **At the weekend do something different, such as going for a walk on the beach or to the park.** Exercise is all about changing our habits and there is nothing to say that it can't be enjoyable. Build it into your weekend as well and try to get the whole family or some friends involved.

Chapter five

How diet and lifestyle AFFECT YOUR WEIGHT

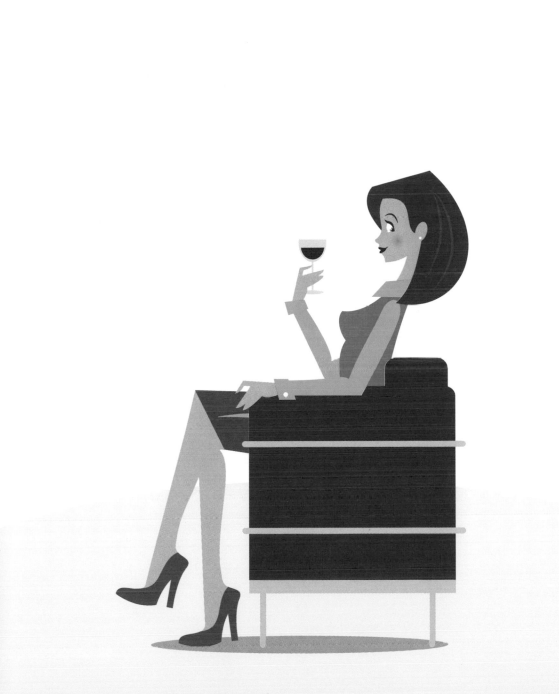

'Education is not preparation for life; education is life itself.' John Dewey

Why crash diets never work

Many women spend huge amounts of money and time on the latest craze diet, which will supposedly make them slim. But rather than deal with the root of the issue, all they are actually doing is dancing around the problem and frustrating themselves in the process. It is a vicious cycle and one that can be hard to break if you have always struggled with your weight.

The most common months for people to begin dieting are January and June. Very often these are 'crash' diets that supposedly enable you to lose weight fast. This is why they appeal to women who are overweight. You've started the new year carrying a few extra pounds or you are getting ready for your summer holiday and feel embarrassed about being seen in a swimming suit. The reality is that the worst thing you can possibly do is experiment with 'yo-yo dieting'. It's not good for your health, your mind or your wellbeing.

For those of you who have experimented with these types of diets, you have probably noticed that the weight always goes back on. Crash diets might give you quick results, but they don't last and they are not the kind of thing you can sustain long term. You are not losing fat when you do a crash diet. Instead, you are just losing muscle mass and water. The reason why the weight doesn't stay off is that you are encouraging your metabolism to slow down. So once the crash diet is finished, you will probably gain the weight back again quite quickly.

Dieting in this way can also leave you feeling quite moody, tired and lacking in energy. You are literally starving your body of the nutrients it needs to function well. We need the right type of food to give us energy. And in terms of our health, we run the risk of weakening our immune system as well. It stands to reason that if you are not eating well, your body will react to that. Iron defiency is something that can be a problem if you are not eating the right types of food. Anaemia could develop, which will leave you feeling lethargic and suffering from bad headaches. Yo-yo dieting over a long period of time can also have more serious consequences. Your vital organs – which include the liver, heart and kidneys – are also being deprived of what they need to work properly.

Crash diets are usually done by women who are in search of a quick-fix solution. The biggest problem I see with this method of weight loss is that the motivation is all wrong. In the long term, you need to be making a lifestyle choice – not constantly searching for the next big fad diet. The psychological effects of crash dieting are really unhealthy as they can have a huge impact on your self-esteem. You are bound to feel disappointed once the results of a crash diet have worn off. Try to view losing weight as your long-term goal, not a temporary solution to get you through to the family wedding in two weeks' time. That will never work. What I did took years, but it paid off. You have to decide to change your ways for good in order to change your body shape.

Where we store fat

Jelly belly, thunder thighs and bingo wings – these are all terms that we ladies jokingly use to refer to our unwanted wobbly bits! We spend so much time looking in the mirror, analysing and agonising over our body shape. We observe our bodies naturally changing over the years as they adjust to pregnancies, the menopause, thyroid problems, etc. – all factors that can contribute to us gaining weight or seeing changes in our body shape. We certainly got the raw deal, didn't we? But do you ever wonder why we store fat in certain places? For some, it all seems to go around the middle area and for others the legs and arms are affected. Fat doesn't usually seem to be evenly distributed when we gain weight. Even when we are on the road to weight loss, there still seem to be areas of our body that are harder to shift the pounds from. I've heard so many women complain about the spare tyre they carry around their middle and how hard it is to lose. Others say that their hips and bum area cause major problems and find it very difficult to get into shape. I remember going to a supermarket once and lifting ten bags of sugar. They were heavy – and I was carrying this weight on my thighs, arms, bum and tummy.

So is there a reason why we store fat in certain places and what does it actually mean? While many people think that their shape and size come down to pure genetics, this is a misconception. I'm sorry to break it to you ladies, but you'll have to stop blaming your mum and dad for this one! Yes, it plays a small role but it turns out it's not all their fault. Research has shown that the fat that collects in certain areas of our body has more to do with our hormones and diet than anything else.

- **Stomach:** Let's start with the stomach, which for so many women is a problem area. Many find that, even when they start to lose weight, their stomach fat seems slower to shift than fat everywhere else. Well, the stomach area may be causing you problems, but your diet may not be totally to blame. It is thought that the weight you gain around this area could be related to stress. When we feel stressed a substance called cortisol is released from our adrenal glands into the body and this causes fat to be deposited around our tummy area. So, if you are stressing over the fact that you are not losing weight here, the chances are that you won't be helping the problem. Much better to focus your energy on eating foods that give the body a chance to get the cortisol balance back to normal levels. And guess what? They are all foods I will be advising you to eat anyway! Cut out all the sugary foods and empty carbohydrates. They will not help the problem area. Instead eat plenty of fish, avocados, beetroot and chicken – anything that contains high levels of lean protein will help.

- **Thighs and bum:** You often hear women describing themselves as being a 'pear' shape, which means that they carry most of their weight around the thigh and bum area. Well, for starters, I'm not a fan of comparing your body shape to fruit! I think we all come in very different shapes and sizes. If you are one of those women who carry weight around this area, it could signify that you have high oestrogen levels. The best thing you can do is try to detoxify the oestrogen by eating a diet that includes vegetables such as cauliflower, cabbage and Brussels sprouts. They might not be to your liking, but they could be the answer to your problems. Once again you have to cut out the processed foods as well and try to eat only natural produce. Also exercise will help. Try doing squats and lunges, which will really focus on the specific area that needs work. The good news is that a study from Oxford University in 2010 showed that women who carry weight on their thigh and bum area are less likely to develop heart disease and type 2 diabetes than those who are heavy around the tummy area.

- **Bingo wings:** Next up we are focusing on those dreaded bingo wings, which really seem to haunt women! A recent study has shown that the cause of this problem area could be related to the toxins found in the plastic bottles we drink from or the plastic containers we eat our lunch out of. The best way to work on this area is through exercise. You need to strengthen the muscles in order to say goodbye to your bingo wings! So, if this is an area that you have been neglecting, it's time to get working. The wings won't go away by themselves and even women who lose weight find they still struggle with them. So try taking up the cross trainer or the rowing machine if you want to banish your bingo wings for good.

The dreaded cellulite

Cellulite even sounds like a scary word, doesn't it? It's certainly something that haunts millions of women all over the world. We have seen the cruel pictures of celebrities with tiny bits of cellulite who have been snapped at an unflattering angle. I'm sure the last thing they need is for such a picture to be plastered all over the front of magazines and papers. But it just goes to show that cellulite happens to us all. The definition of cellulite is 'persistent subcutaneous fat causing dimpling in the skin, especially on women's hips and thighs'. Basically, it is excess fat and toxins that become lodged under the skin. The fibres become hard and the fat is compressed, which causes a rippled or unsmooth look. Unfortunately women are the victims when it comes to cellulite, while men get away without it! In fact, it would be very rare for a man to have cellulite. Hormonal changes that women go through in their lifetime, such as during pregnancy and menopause, play a role in cellulite. Even slim women find they can develop it. It is estimated that over 85 per cent of women suffer from cellulite at some point. We all have a certain amount of fat on our bodies, so we are all susceptible to it. Cellulite is something we can blame on our genes, however, and many people find it runs in the family. So if your mum has cellulite, it's likely that you could develop it too.

I always think that it's better to know the facts – that way you can deal with the problem. As you get older and your skin becomes thinner, you are more prone to developing cellulite. Also, when you lose weight you might find that your cellulite appears to be worse than before. This happens because your skin

It is estimated that over 85 per cent of women suffer from cellulite at some point.

Know the facts – that way you can deal with the problem.

becomes looser as it sheds the pounds. Cellulite develops primarily on our thighs and hips because the enzyme lipoprotein lipase transports fat to tissues around the body. Apart from these areas, it can also be found on the stomach and bottom. Often it is a real cause of upset for women and many find that it affects their confidence. Take comfort in the fact that you are not on your own; it's just one of those things you have to contend with. The bad news is that there is no wonderful, instant cure for cellulite, although there are steps you can take to try to reduce its appearance.

Here are my top tips to help you deal with cellulite:

- **Give yourself a massage:** Time for some pampering, ladies, as one of the things known to improve the appearance of cellulite is a good massage. Treat yourself every couple of months. Massaging the affected area is said to help improve circulation and also get rid of trapped toxins in the body. This makes it possible to break down the cellulite and ultimately make the skin smoother.

- **Avoid processed, fatty, sugary and fried foods:** They do not do cellulite any favours, so avoiding these is essential. These are the foods that cause the accumulation of fat and toxins underneath our skin. Good food will help to break down these deposits, so it is possible to get rid of them. Going forward, keep in mind the importance of detoxing and cleansing your body of the build-up.

- **Cut down on coffee, fizzy drinks and alcohol:** These all contribute towards the build-up of toxins in our body and can lead to cellulite. When you drink coffee and alcohol, your body can become dehydrated and in turn your fat cells hold on to more liquid. As a result these cells begin to swell up under the skin and appear as cellulite. Water and herbal teas are always the best options.

- **Eat more fruit, vegetables and foods containing fibre:** These are all great for getting toxins out of your system.

- **Exercise regularly:** This can really help cellulite, especially any physical activity that involves fat burning. Try doing a level of cardiovascular exercise to get your heart rate up. Cardio exercise is the one that burns calories and this is what you need. Running and cycling are good examples. Also squats are great as they concentrate on the specific area where cellulite occurs.

- **Limit your salt intake:** Salt contributes to the build-up of toxins in the body, which in turn leads to cellulite.

- **Drink plenty of water:** This will help to flush out your system and also keep you hydrated. The amount you need to drink every day depends on a number of factors, including size, how physically active you are and what the temperature is. We obviously need more water during hot weather to stay hydrated. On average it is recommended that we drink eight glasses or 1.2 litres of water every day.

- **Quit smoking:** If you smoke and suffer from cellulite, it's time to quit. People who smoke are likely to find that their skin ages more quickly than others', because smoking assists in the breakdown of collagen. This in turn leads to your skin becoming thinner at a younger age, making cellulite more apparent.

- **Cover up:** If all else fails, avoid wearing clothes that draw attention to the area. There is no point exposing an area that makes you feel uncomfortable. We all have body hang-ups and if cellulite is yours, cover that area by dressing cleverly, also wear good foundation.

If you smoke and suffer from cellulite, it's time to quit.

People who spend the day seated at a desk are unlikely to lose weight.

How your job and lifestyle can affect your weight

According to the World Health Organisation, obesity levels have nearly doubled since 1980. A government study in the US carried out by the Centers for Disease Control and Prevention found that nearly 80 per cent of adult Americans do not get the recommended amounts of exercise each week. And a report published by the *Lancet* medical journal showed that in the UK 63.3 per cent of adults (with higher rates in women than in men) do not meet recommended amounts of activity.

It stands to reason that people who spend eight hours of the day seated at a desk are unlikely to lose weight while doing so. Perhaps we have become a lazy nation, but how feasible is it to spend a greater proportion of the day in an upright position?

Like it or hate it, if you're one of the thousands of women and men all over the country who spend your day sitting down, you are at risk of falling victim to what is now being referred to as 'desk derrière!' Yes, you read right. There is a serious downside to the office job. A survey, which was done by Tel Aviv University, scanned the buttocks of people who are inactive on a regular basis and found that their muscles were shrinking and breaking down due to a lack of exercise. This was leading to thick layers of fat building up around the area, which deposited itself deep inside the muscle tissue. There, you have the facts!

Not moving around during the day will affect not only your bum area, but also your hips and thighs. What happens is that your hip flexor muscle, which is at the front of the hip, can start to tighten when you spend too much time sitting at a desk. The unfortunate fact is that, while it can affect both women and men, women are actually more likely to develop problems with fat in this area. This is because of lipoprotein lipase (see page 60), which appears in much higher levels in women than in men. As women, we store more fat around the hips. It seems unfair, but that's just the way it is. Once again we get a raw deal!

Hairdressers and shop workers should be very happy with the latest research carried out by a doctor at the University of Chester. The research claims that by standing for three hours of every day you will burn off 8lb of fat per year. Maybe it doesn't sound like a huge amount, but when you are trying to lose weight it's fair to say that every little counts.

Combating the effects of an office job

If you have a job that leaves you confined to your desk for most of the day, here is what you can do to avoid the dreaded 'desk derrière':

- **Get moving:** The first thing to do is to get the idea of 'moving more regularly' into your head. Put on a pair of runners and try walking to and from work; you will be much more likely to walk at a pace and with purpose if you are wearing the correct footwear. It might not be the fashion trend of the century, but it will help to keep you fit. If you drive to work, force yourself to leave your car a fair distance from your workplace and walk the last bit of the journey. Usually when we search for a parking space we look for one that is as close as possible to our destination. Now is the moment to change the habits of a lifetime and reap the benefits of being a little more active.

- **Change your habits:** When you arrive at work in the morning, take the stairs and not the lift if you have a choice. By taking the stairs, you are getting your muscles moving at the start of the day. It's all about habit and not always taking the lazy option!

- **Don't stay at your desk all day:** Try to move around as often as you can during the day, as it will help to get your muscles moving. If you spend a lot of the day on the phone, get yourself a cordless model. Make sure you leave your desk at lunchtime, even if it's just to take a stroll around the office. While you are sitting at your desk, get into the habit of stretching your legs and arms as much as you can – forget the fact that you might look silly; instead focus on your goal which is to combat the ill effects of a desk job.

Failing to prepare is preparing to fail!

- **Drink plenty of water:** I might sound like a broken record now, but drinking water is crucial here. Dehydration leads to you feeling tired and lacking in energy, which means that you are more inclined to look for a pick-me-up in the form of a sugary snack.

- **Bring a packed lunch:** This way you are in total control of what you are eating and therefore less likely to take the unhealthy option. You know already that cutting out the junk food will help your situation, but there is no harm in reminding you. Don't be tempted by the lure of vending machines and office canteens. Stay strong and stick to what you know works best for you. You know my motto, 'Failing to prepare is preparing to fail!'

- **Exercise regularly:** For those of you who are confined to a desk during the week, it's so important that you exercise regularly – and I mean at least three times a week. Remember that you are already at a disadvantage because you don't have the liberty of moving about regularly with your day job, so you have to make up for it as much as possible at other times. At the weekends, make sure that you get out for a walk. Not only is walking good exercise, but also it's great for clearing your head. Don't underestimate housework. If you give your house a serious clean once a week, you are on your feet and exercising without realising. The result is a spotless home and extra calories burnt. If a workout or exercising is proving tough, take a day off, close the curtains, put on your favourite music and have a good old-fashioned boogie in the comfort of your home. Dancing at high energy is a fantastic way of staying fit. Just ask Kelly Osbourne, who attributes some of her weight loss to being a keen dancer.

- **Take time to play with your children:** When we lead a busy life we often forget to take time out to play and have fun. Get a ball, go outside into your garden or even the park and run around for half an hour. Not only are you encouraging your children to be more active, but also you are burning calories yourself.

How food affects your mood

We all know that junk food, processed food and fatty foods are not good for our health or our waistline. However, is it possible that eating the wrong kind of food also has a negative effect on our mood? You often hear people saying that when they are eating healthily that they feel much better about themselves and are also in a more positive frame of mind. So how does food affect our mood and what should we be eating to stay happy?

- **Sugar:** Unless it's in a natural form, sugar is best avoided. Food and drinks containing high levels of 'refined sugar' interfere with the blood sugar in your body. They provide you with an instant rush and leave you with the crash when the effect has worn off, which is exactly what happens with fizzy drinks. Much better to switch to natural fruit juices instead. Any of the citrus fruits such as lemon, orange or grapefruit are good options because they contain vitamin C, which is known for helping to reduce stress. Grape juice is also a good source of natural sugar, as well as being rich in antioxidants. If you're a strawberry fan, it's good news, because this fruit produces endorphins, which are said to put you in a better mood. Bananas, which are rich in potassium and fibre, are also great for relieving stress.

- **Coffee and tea:** I don't know about you, but I am one of those people who enjoy my coffee first thing in the morning. It helps set me up for the day, it's a habit I've formed and something I wouldn't be without. In fact, I don't think I'd work properly if I didn't have that morning fix! The thing about coffee is that it's fine to drink it in moderation, but if you drink it constantly to boost your mood it is unlikely to work – in fact, it can leave you feeling in a negative mood. If this happens, try switching to tea. Tea contains natural antioxidants and it is also known to relieve stress and make you feel calm. Green tea is better again as it contains even less caffeine.

We need a certain amount of carbs in our diet, but not the 'empty' variety.

- **Carbs:** We all need a certain amount of carbohydrates in our diet, but what we don't need is the 'empty' variety – for example, those found in cakes, pastries, white bread and bagels, etc. The list is endless, but let's just say it's all the things that are bad for us! I remember grabbing a bagel once when I was hungry and needed energy. Well, I reached for the wrong food. Not long after eating it I felt sluggish and completely unmotivated. Try to switch to wholegrain or complex carbohydrates instead, such as those provided by brown bread or brown rice; they take longer to digest and therefore don't leave you with a crash after eating them. They provide more nutrients than 'empty' carbs, and yet there is still a certain comfort gained from eating them.

- **Nuts and seeds:** We have established that snacking on sugary and processed foods will not leave us feeling happy, so what can we eat when we need a lift? Well, nuts are a great option. These are filled with vitamin E and magnesium, both of which are great for boosting your mood, and nuts also provide energy. Another benefit of eating nuts is they encourage the production of serotonin, a feel-good brain chemical – in particular, walnuts and pecan nuts contain high serotonin levels; or you could choose almonds, walnuts or cashews to reap the benefits. Next time you have a sugar craving, be prepared. Have some nuts in your handbag to give you a lift.

- **Omega-3s:** In recent years, there have been many studies done to try to understand whether or not there is a link between depression and diet. Experts claim that people who suffer with depression need to make sure that their diet is rich in omega-3 fatty acids, which we know are found in oily fish. Next time your mood needs a lift, try bringing out the mackerel, salmon, tuna or sardines, which are all full of omega-3. Or if you are vegetarian, reach for the tofu, soya beans or Brussels sprouts.

- **Water:** Dehydration can be one of the most common reasons why people find themselves in a low mood. Not drinking enough water every day can leave you tired and lacking in energy. You have to keep your body hydrated. Carrying that water bottle everywhere you go makes it easier to get into the habit of drinking more. If you don't believe me, take it from Jennifer Anniston who last year claimed that not drinking enough water makes you cranky!

It's clear that there is a link between the foods we eat and our mood. So if you've been feeling tired, grumpy or stressed, it's good to know that there is a possible solution. I always think that it comes down to making a choice. Life is hectic enough without being in a bad mood, so take control of it by controlling your diet.

How poor diet affects your sleep

Many of us take for granted the ability to get a good night's sleep. I'm talking about the kind of sleep that allows you to wake up feeling refreshed and ready for the day ahead. I try to get my eight hours every night – it means I function better and, when I'm on the go, it's a necessity. However, what you may not realise is that being overweight can have an impact on both your sleep patterns and the quality of your sleep.

The foods we eat play a role in how we sleep. If your daily diet comprises foods that are high in sugar or caffeine, it's only natural that you are going to find it hard to switch off when you go to bed at night. There is a reason why it's not advisable to give children too many sweets! This pattern becomes a vicious circle because what happens to many people after a bad night's sleep is that they wake up feeling they need caffeine to give them a kick. As the day goes on and tiredness sets in, their need for a sugar rush increases. Then the crash comes and the damage has been done in terms of gaining weight. If this sounds familiar, something needs to change.

Ways to ensure you get a good night's rest:
- **Eating well:** If you want to get a good night's sleep, it is essential that you eat well during the day. Fill up on foods that are rich in nutrients and keep your brain active during the day, so it doesn't keep you active during the small hours.

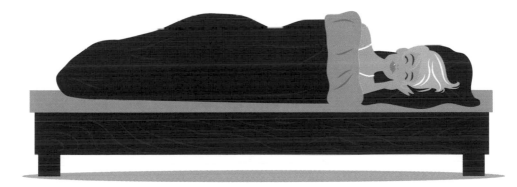

There is a terrible misconception that if you smoke more you will eat less.

- **Limit your caffeine intake:** Try to limit the amount of coffee and caffeinated drinks you have every day as this can play havoc with sleep patterns. Do not drink coffee after 3pm.

- **Regulate your meal times:** Leave at least three hours after eating before you go to bed. And avoid anything that is high in fat or sugar last thing at night. These foods are hard to digest, which means that if you eat them in the evening they are more likely to be stored as fat. Studies have shown that there is a definite link between people who have fatty diets and those who suffer from sleep deprivation.

- **Exercise during the day:** Exercise is essential if you really want to feel the benefit of a good night's sleep. It helps to burn energy earlier in the day, which means that when you go to bed at night you are ready to fall asleep. If you can get a workout early in the morning, it's a great way to start the day. Not only is exercise a good stress reliever, but it also helps to put you in a better mood for what's to come. Many people only have time to exercise after work, which is fine; however, just make sure you leave a couple hours in between your workout and going to bed. This should give your body a chance to wind down.

Smoking

When you are making changes in your life that include becoming fit and healthy, it stands to reason that smoking plays no part. There is a terrible misconception that if you smoke more you will eat less. Maybe this is true for some people who already have an unhealthy lifestyle, but for many smoking goes hand in hand with poor diet, overeating and lack of exercise. This combination is what contributes to people putting on weight; if it becomes a way of life, the habit becomes even harder to break.

If you are overweight and a smoker, your chances of developing heart disease are greatly increased. You are putting a huge amount of pressure on your heart, which is the single most important muscle in your body. Toxins build up in your body when you are a regular smoker. Your arteries become clogged and this can increase your blood pressure. Obviously being overweight as well means you are putting yourself at even more risk. It's fair to say that most people know this and yet it is still not enough to encourage them to quit once and for all.

Every decision you make in relation to your weight will be your own. But think about it in terms of the bigger picture. Being fit and healthy in your every-day life just will not work if you continue to smoke. How could you possibly imagine it would? Think about the effect smoking has on your heart and how you are potentially putting your life at risk. As dramatic as that sounds, it's true. Whatever your situation is, you owe it to yourself to stop smoking and give yourself every chance to be in the best possible shape you can.

Do not use the fear of gaining weight and slipping into bad habits as an excuse for you not to give up. If it is or has been your way of thinking, let it go, because at the end of the day cigarettes could kill you. That's the reality that you need to face up to. The message that you need to get inside your head is, 'Weight can be lost, lungs cannot.'

Here are my tips if you are struggling to quit smoking:

1. **Spring clean:** Clear the house of cigarettes and ashtrays. You don't need constant reminders of smoking when you are trying to move on. If you feel there is still a cigarette smell in the house, do a little spring clean and get rid of it. New beginnings and a new you.

2. **Find the motivation:** As when deciding to lose weight, you need to discover what your motivation to give up smoking really is. What is driving you to quit? What is your main focus? Be clear why you want to quit. Write down your reasons and try to re-enforce them every day.

3. **Avoid any temptation:** Keep away from situations that trigger your desire to smoke. For some, people it's having a drink. So you may need to cut back on the alcohol for a while. For many people, alcohol can really encourage their smoking habit. If you are serious about giving up, you will have to make sacrifices.

4. **Be prepared:** If you feel that you are craving a cigarette and are tempted to reach for the wrong food to fight it, be prepared. You will crave a cigarette – it's inevitable. Have a healthy snack on hand.

5. **Move more:** You should find that exercise gets easier as you begin to lose weight and it's worth noting that exercise is essential if you are giving up cigarettes. It helps the body to fight the nicotine cravings. If you feel a craving coming on, grab your runners and get outside. It's so important to keep active.

6. **Avoid stress:** You may feel stressed during the first few weeks of quitting, so do the best you can to manage that. Go for a massage or sit down and watch a film to switch off. Learn to listen to your body so that you can recognise the signs of feeling stressed.

7. **Don't give in:** You might have days when you are tempted to give in because you think your goal seems impossible. Whatever you do, keep going. If you do slip up, forget it and move on. Tomorrow is another day, so be patient.

The demon drink

Once the weekend comes I love to relax and have a couple of glasses of wine. It's my way of de-stressing after a busy week and it's definitely one of my favourite times. Comfy clothes, glass of white wine in my hand and something I love on the television… or the fire lit and my favourite music on. It's the little things in life that are important, isn't it? There is nothing to say that being healthy can't involve enjoying a drink or two. I'm a big believer in time out, where we switch off and have a little rest. We all need it, as life can get a bit crazy now and then.

Losing weight definitely had an impact on what I drank. Gone were the rum and sugar-laden cokes – or in other words a recipe for disaster! So how many calories do different drinks contain? And what effect does alcohol have on weight loss?

Unlike food and drink, alcohol doesn't actually need digesting, so it is processed into the body quite quickly. Therefore it plays havoc with our metabolism. When we drink our body becomes focused solely on trying to process the alcohol, the result being that any food that is already in our system becomes harder to digest. Instead of the food being broken down properly, it is stored as fat. This is where one of the first problems arises when it comes to having a drink and trying to lose weight.

A good night's sleep is not something you will get if you have had a drink. You may think that you are sleeping soundly, but it's not deep sleep. After drinking alcohol you may find that you go straight to sleep, but you will skip the first stage, known as REM (rapid eye movement). So you'll find that even if you sleep for a full eight hours you feel tired and sluggish the next day. The more you drink before you go to bed at night, the more disrupted your sleep is likely to be. You'll end up feeling drained of energy and find it hard to get motivated. This could impact on your weight loss if you're tired and struggling to make healthy food choices. You will also find it much harder to exercise, as your body feels so tired.

Drinking tips for people who are trying to lose weight:

- **Time your food carefully:** A good tip is to have your meal a few hours before you plan to have a drink. That way, you are giving your food plenty of time to digest, which means that the alcohol won't have as much of an effect.

- **Don't skip meals:** Alcohol has no nutritional value and should not be substituted for a meal. Forget the idea of trying to save on calories if you are going out for the night. All that will happen is that when you do eat again your body will immediately store the food as fat.

- **Everything in moderation:** In the same way as you practise portion control when it comes to food, try to become more aware of drink measurements when it comes to alcohol (see page 72).

- **Drink plenty of water:** Alcohol is a diuretic, which means that it can cause dehydration – a fact that many of you are probably aware of, having woken up feeling thirsty the morning after the night before. To avoid dehydration, try to get into the habit of sipping water when you are drinking alcohol – that way, you will tend not to drink as much of the latter. If you do suffer from a hangover the following morning, stick to water: it's the best thing for rehydrating your body and it has no calories! (See pages 115–116 for more hangover cures.)

Forget trying to save on calories if you are going out for the night.

- **Don't reach for the fast food:** The reason you often feel hungry after having a few drinks is that alcohol lowers your blood-sugar levels. So what happens is you end up eating a lot more than you normally would and possibly making the wrong food choices. Alcohol provides you with nothing but empty calories. If you reach for fast food at the end of a night out, there will be only one outcome! Everything that you eat will be stored immediately as fat.

Alcohol facts

If you are armed with the facts, you are more likely to make the right choices. The most important thing you need to know about alcohol in terms of losing weight is what it contains:

- **Wine** – a 175ml glass contains about 130 calories.

- **Beer** – a pint contains about 190 calories.

- **Champagne/sparkling wine/Prosecco** – a 125ml glass contains about 95 calories.

- **Vodka** – a single measure (25ml) and a 'full-fat' soft drink contains about 108 calories; a single measure (25ml) and a 'diet' soft drink contains about 54 calories.

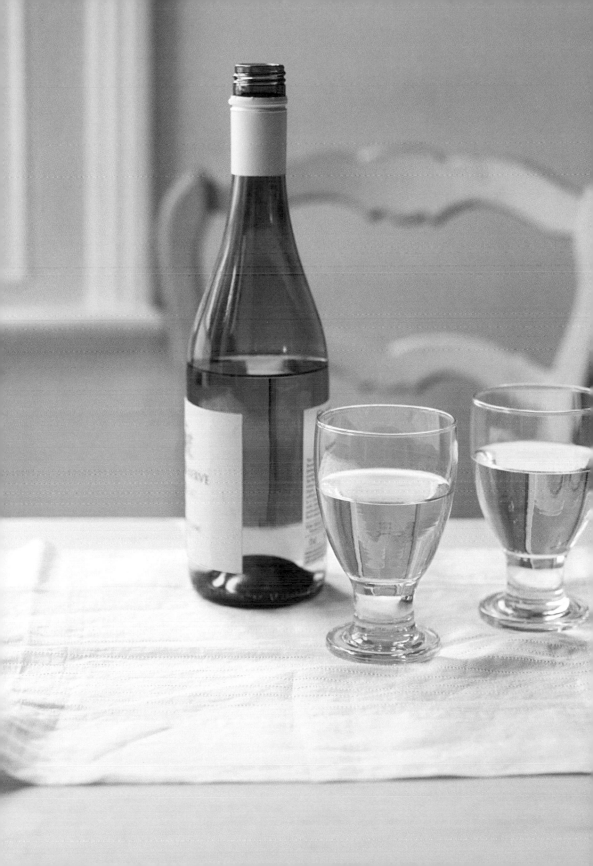

Chapter six

What makes
A BALANCED DIET

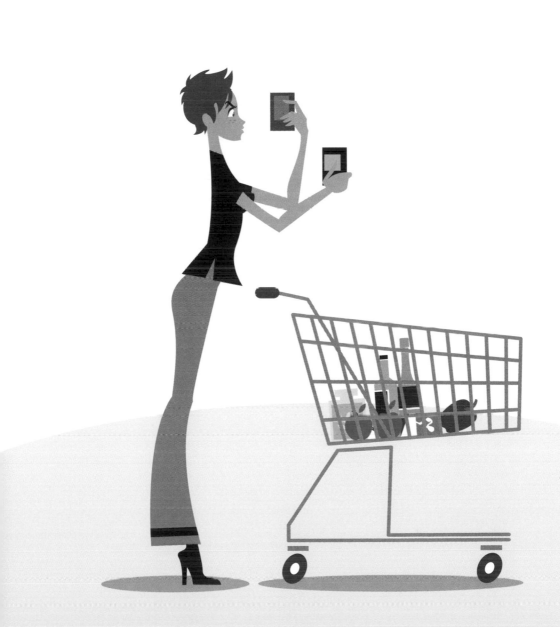

'To eat is a necessity, but to eat intelligently is an art.' La Rochefoucauld

When I cast my mind back to my days of breakfast rolls and endless packets of biscuits, I wonder whether there was a single ounce of nutritional value in my daily diet. I wrote earlier about the celebrity culture that we are now exposed to and how it has definitely made women more aware of reading food labels and constantly avoiding foods that are high in fat. For me, eating well is about striking a balance and I think that over the years I have learned how to do that. I have retrained my brain to appreciate what I am putting inside my body. Real food such as fruit, vegetables, fresh fish and meat doesn't need labels. It is nutritious and over time you will find that eating a balanced diet has an impact on not only your health but also your emotional wellbeing.

What is a balanced diet?

In simple terms, a balanced diet means eating the right amount of food to coincide with how active you are, as well as eating a wide variety of foods – including fruit, vegetables, wholegrains, dairy, meat, fish, beans or pulses and eggs. If you are a vegetarian, your diet should include plenty of nuts, seeds, eggs, dairy, beans, fruit, vegetables and wholegrains. When you see the different foods listed like this, eating well seems quite straightforward, and yet the daily lure of the wrong foods can often override our best intentions. The most useful thing I ever did was to learn about the various foods that should make up our daily diet. Once you have that information, and it is instilled in you, eating well should become a way of life. Let me go through with you in simple terms the variety of foods we should be eating to keep us healthy.

Grains and starchy foods

Starchy foods such as bread, cereals, rice and pasta are all a good source of energy and the main source of a range of nutrients in our diet. As well as starch, these foods contain fibre, calcium, iron and B vitamins. As a rule of thumb, it's always best to choose the wholegrain versions, which are higher in fibre than white bread, white rice or white pasta. From a weight-loss point of view, the advantage of eating wholegrain foods that are high in fibre is they help you feel full for longer, which means you are less likely to snack.

Protein

Foods such as poultry, red meat, eggs, fish, seeds, nuts and pulses are a good source of protein, B vitamins and minerals such as zinc and iron. We need protein for growth and cell repair, and we need iron to prevent us from becoming anaemic. Be aware that some meat can be quite high in fat, so where possible choose lean cuts. If you are vegetarian, you can get your recommended daily intake of protein from eggs, nuts and beans or pulses.

Dairy produce

This includes milk, yogurt and cheese. Dairy products are a good source of protein, but they are also rich in calcium, which is needed for building strong bones and teeth. To enjoy the health benefits of dairy food without eating too much fat, choose semi-skimmed milk and low-fat cheese or yogurt – however, be aware that some low-fat products contain even more sugar than the full-fat version, making them less beneficial. For more on this, refer to the labels of individual products to see if the low-fat version is worthwhile. Note that research has shown that lowering the fat content does not reduce the calcium content. For more information on fat, see page 78.

Fruit and vegetables

Fruit and vegetables are a vital source of vitamins and minerals, which play an important role in helping to prevent infection. They are also a good natural source of dietary fibre, which is important in helping food move through the digestive system. We all know that it is important to get at least five portions of fruit and vegetables every day, but this doesn't mean a big change to your diet (see page 121). A piece of fruit is the perfect alternative to a sugary snack as it is rich in natural sugar but fat-free. It is thought that eating plenty of fruit and veg may help reduce the risk of certain diseases such as heart disease, type 2 diabetes and obesity.

Understanding fats

There is often the misconception that all fat is bad for you, and it should be removed altogether from your diet, but this is not entirely true. In fact, we all need some fat in our diet because it helps the body absorb certain nutrients. The important thing to bear in mind is that some fats are good for you and others are bad.

When looking at the amount of fat in your diet, you should focus on reducing the proportion of saturated fat. Remember, we don't need to cut down on every type of fat. Certain fats, such as the unsaturated fats found in oily fish, are really good for you.

Good fats: unsaturated fats

Eating unsaturated fat instead of saturated fat can help to lower blood cholesterol, which can reduce the risk of heart disease. There are two types of unsaturated fat, monounsaturated and polyunsaturated.

- **Monounsaturated fats** are found in a number of foods and oils, such as olive oil, nuts, avocados and olives.
- **Polyunsaturated fats**, otherwise known as 'essential fatty acids', include omega-3 and omega-6. Omega-3 fatty acids are found in most fish, in particular in oily fish such as mackerel, trout and herring, as well as in tuna and salmon. If you are worried you are not getting your daily allowance, I can highly recommend a fish oil supplement. Omega 6 is found in most vegetable oils and nuts, in particular walnuts and almonds.

Bear in mind that some fats are good for you and others are bad.

Learn to understand labels to see how much sugar and fat a product contains.

Bad fats: saturated and trans fats

- **Saturated fats** are found in animal products such as meat and dairy. Foods high in saturated fat include meat produce, such as sausages and pies, as well as dairy produce, such as butter, cheese, cream and ice cream. Saturated fats are known to raise blood cholesterol, which can increase your risk of heart disease, so these fats are best kept to a minimum.
- **Trans fats** are often considered to be the worst type. Like saturated fats, trans fats raise cholesterol in the blood. Trans fats are found in processed foods containing hydrogenated vegetable oil, such as margarine, ready meals, crisps, sauces, pies and pastries. By law, hydrogenated vegetable oil must appear on the ingredients label if it is present in the food, so it is important to familiarise yourself with food labels in order to know what you are buying. Be aware that trans fats can go under different names, such as 'partially hydrogenated vegetable oil'.

Myths about food labelling

Learning to understand labels is necessary to see how much sugar and fat a product contains. Cutting out refined produce is definitely the way to go. It is always better to buy foods in their natural form as this is the only way of ensuring that they have not been filled with additives, including MSG. The shocking fact is that so many processed foods contain far more fat and sugar than our recommended daily intake. So while you might think the calories seem reasonable, these other items could be more damaging.

Sometimes we are misled into thinking that certain foods are good for us, when in fact they are not. Very often we are taken in by clever advertising or confusing labelling; however, just because a label declares a food is 'fat-free' or 'low in fat' it doesn't mean it's healthy – these versions often contain far more calories in the form of sugar. Clever labelling and hidden ingredients such as preservatives and sweeteners fool people on a daily basis.

Good for you or bad for you?

In this section I want to open your eyes so that you can learn to recognise which foods are healthy and which ones to avoid.

- **Health bars and cereal bars:** Not all of these bars are off-limits, but their labelling can certainly be misleading. Often health bars are sold as an alternative to junk food, so if you are trying to stick to a healthy diet they might seem like a good option. However, it always pays to check the label before you buy; if the fat and sugar content are high, a piece of fruit might be a better option. Ideally you should be looking for a health bar that contains less than 5g fat, preferably with plenty of fibre. Make sure that the calorie content is not too high – anything over 150kcal is on the high side. If in doubt, you can always make your own healthy version using the recipe on page 138. Note that these bars are not a substitute for other foods in your diet and shouldn't replace lunch or dinner.

- **Diet drinks:** You pick up a can of diet cola thinking it's absolutely fine, but what you may not know is that a number of studies have revealed that people who consume diet drinks on a regular basis have a higher risk of becoming overweight or obese. Diet drinks contain artificial sweeteners, which are actually far sweeter than those used in regular soft drinks. Artificial sweeteners are responsible for tricking your body into thinking that you are getting sugar. You, in turn, crave more and find yourself feeling hungry. They also slow down your metabolism, meaning you burn fewer calories. While more research needs to be carried out in this area, there is no doubt that you could be drinking something far healthier if you stuck to homemade fruit juices or water. And if that is not reason enough to shun them, diet drinks contain absolutely no nutritional value. Carrying a bottle of water in your handbag is definitely the way to go!

- **Fruit juices:** When made at home these can be a really healthy option. However, if you are buying a carton be aware that many contain added sugar and some manufacturers also remove the fruit pulp, which is where all the goodness is. My advice is to buy a juicer and make your own. Of course, even homemade juice is high in sugar, so it should be enjoyed in moderation. If you have to buy from the supermarket, make sure you choose a 'not from concentrate' type, with no added water, sugar or preservatives.

- **Bread:** If it's white, don't bite! You will have heard this saying time and time again, but have you removed white bread from your diet? If the answer is no, I hope I can convince you! White bread is made from refined white flour, which contains minimal amounts of nutrients and fibre. It also has a high sugar and salt content. White bread is often referred to as an 'empty' carbohydrate, which means it has no place in your food plan. You need to replace it with wholegrain bread, which is far healthier. Many people find it hard to imagine a day without white bread, but if you are serious about changing your lifestyle you should eliminate it from your diet now. To avoid temptation, don't have it in the house. No excuses – just get rid of it!

- **Salad dressing:** While the salad you are eating is healthy, the dressing that goes with it is more than likely not. This applies to dressings that are shop-bought and the ones you are served while eating out. Most contain refined oils, which means that any goodness has been removed. If you want to be sure that your salad is healthy, always make your own dressing (see page 144 for a recipe).

It may sound simple, but cutting back on the amount of food on your plate will make it much easier to eat less!

Understanding calories

In simple terms, there are two types of calories – those that provide you with energy and those that will leave you raiding the fridge again not long after you've eaten. Most people could happily eat their recommended daily amount of calories and still find themselves hungry if they didn't eat the right sort of foods.

You get the good type of calories from fruit and vegetables, which contain plenty of fibre. Fibre is a great way of consuming calories as it keeps you feeling fuller for longer, which in turn prevents you from reaching for something you shouldn't. Protein-rich foods such as chicken, fish and lentils are also great. When it comes to calories some foods take more energy to digest than others, so once again make wise choices. You don't want foods that can be digested too easily as these are more likely to be stored as fat. High-sugar foods break down quickly, leaving you hungry again a short period after eating. Always opt for wholegrain versions instead.

The other way to control the calories is to practise portion control. It may sound simple, but cutting back on the amount of food on your plate will make it much easier to eat less! This is harder to do when you are eating out as you can't control the serving, but be sensible when choosing and don't be tempted by the option you know is bound to contain more calories and fat.

Many takeaway and fast-food meals contain more than your recommended daily allowance of calories in one serving, which is slightly scary but true. A large popcorn in the cinema can contain up to 2000 calories!

Should we count calories?

This is one of the diet dilemmas that many women spend hours deliberating over, and the debate is ongoing. How many calories are in a cupcake? If I don't have a starter, can I eat the carbonara? Are there more calories in a latte or a cappuccino? We torture ourselves wondering how many calories certain foods contain to the point where it can become an unhealthy obsession. But is it helpful for us to try constantly to account for every single ounce of food that passes our lips?

Over the years we have been led to believe that the fewer calories we consume, the more likely we are to stay slim. Yes, there is an element of truth in this, but what is often overlooked is that calories are not the only things that count. When trying to implement a healthy and balanced diet we need to be aware of the fat and sugar content in the foods we eat as well. These are actually the things that cause us to gain weight in the first place, not the calories alone. The recommended daily calorie intake is 2500 for men and 2000 for women, depending on age and level of activity. There is no secret to weight loss and being fixated on calories will not help unless you are also armed with the other tools you need. It's all about food awareness – learning which foods are nutritious and retraining your brain to make positive food choices.

The truth about your metabolism

Here is something that always gets me thinking and I doubt I'll be alone on this one. Why can some of my skinny friends eat bread, have a good metabolism and not put on weight? It doesn't seem fair! During the week I avoid bread, as I know that it will immediately make me bloated. At weekends, I always treat myself to some brown bread, but never white. It just does not suit me and I know straight away that I'll feel awful afterwards. It shocks me when I meet women who say they can eat it every day. Is there some kind of secret club that I don't know about? Are these women superhuman? Well, of course I know they're not, but I am probably just a tiny bit jealous! When you hear someone boast about their ultra-fast metabolism, what exactly does it mean and is it possible to change yours?

In order to understand why our metabolism can be fast or slow we need to find out how it actually works. Your metabolism is a biochemical process that is in charge of turning what you eat into nutrients. It then decides what fat can be stored and what waste it can get rid of. You have probably already heard of the basic metabolic rate, which describes how fast or slowly your body breaks down your food. This rate is responsible for what kind of metabolism you have and ultimately what you weigh. Therefore, when you hear people talk about having a fast metabolism these are usually the ones who find it easier to lose or maintain weight.

Those who live on a sugary and high-fat diet are much more likely to have a slow metabolism.

If you feel that you fall into the category of slow metabolism, do not despair.

Research has shown that genetics play a very small role in what kind of metabolism you have, so this should not be used as an excuse – I've lost count of the number of women I've heard say that their mothers have big bones, hips, thighs, etc. If you are lucky enough to have a fast metabolism and are not prone to putting on weight, it's important that you try to maintain a healthy diet as much as you can. Even though your weight might be fine now, it is always possible for poor diet to play havoc with your system – you've been warned!

If you feel that you fall into the category of slow metabolism, do not despair. To some extent you can change whether it is fast or slow. Those who live on a sugary and high-fat diet are much more likely to have a slow metabolism. So what you eat every day does contribute towards it. Don't suddenly go and starve yourself, as we know this will have a negative effect on your weight. Do, however, try to switch the bad foods for something that is better for you.

How to kickstart a slow metabolism
If you know you have a slow metabolism, there are some ways to kickstart it into action:

- **Always eat breakfast:** If you skip this meal in the morning, your body will go into starvation mode and store fat. The consequences are that your metabolism will slow down even further.

- **Drink plenty of water:** Dehydration will slow down your metabolism further. A study published in Germany in 2003 showed that drinking 17 fluid ounces of water a day (which is approximately 500ml) boosted the subjects' metabolic rate by 30 per cent. This is proof that drinking water throughout the day is a must.

- **Switch to green tea:** This is said to have properties that kickstart the metabolism.

- **Eat plenty of raw vegetables**, such as carrots, broccoli, tomatoes and spinach. These vegetables take longer to digest and therefore require more energy, which also helps to speed up your metabolism.

- **Eat more spicy food:** Spices are thought to boost your metabolism temporarily, which is good for preventing overeating. They also give you that full feeling. Try adding spicy pepper or some chilli to your omelette or stir-fry.

- **Exercise regularly:** This is essential for people with a slow metabolism, whose thyroid gland often doesn't work as hard. Try to do something like running or swimming, which are both really effective for burning calories. Brisk walking is also beneficial. If you have a desk job, try to move around regularly throughout the day – or at least stand up and stretch your body every hour or so. Small changes will go a long way in helping you to speed up that metabolism.

The truth about salt

It is all too easy to become obsessed with fat content and calorie counting when we are trying to lose weight, yet the road to a healthier lifestyle comes down to us becoming knowledgeable about all aspects of the foods we eat. One of the most talked-about ingredients in recent years has been salt. Many experts have told us to cut it out completely because it has no nutritional value, resulting in us steering clear of the saltshaker at all costs. The truth is that we all need some salt in our diet but, as with many things, too much of it is a bad thing. If your diet is high in salt, you run the risk of developing high blood pressure, which in turn could lead to more serious problems such as heart disease and stroke. Years ago, we never seemed to have this problem – everyone used to put a little mound of salt on the

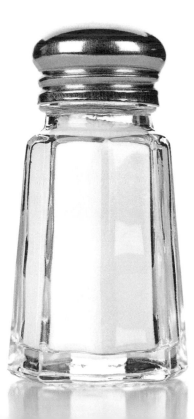

side of their plate when they were eating a meal – but that was because food wasn't processed back then. The main problem that we face today is that most of the foods we purchase in the supermarket are processed. Processed foods are notorious for containing far more than the recommended daily intake of salt. On average, an adult should be consuming no more than 4g (under a teaspoon) of salt per day.

How to cut down on salt

Cutting down on salt in your diet isn't an impossible task; you just have to be aware of where the hidden salt lies.

- Take your time in the supermarket and be aware of foods that have high levels (see below). Keep it in your mind that all processed foods contain large amounts of salt, as does fast food, so once again there is a good reason for making your meals from scratch.
- Where possible, buy meat from your local butcher as it is less likely to be injected with as much salt as the vacuum-packed variety.
- When cooking at home, eliminate salt and switch to herbs and spices. Pepper and chillies are a great way of adding flavour to a meal.
- Make any sauces or dressings yourself to ensure that the salt content is kept to a minimum; those bought in jars can be particularly high in salt.

Top 10 salty foods

1 **Bread:** For all you bread lovers out there, it's bad news. Bread is one of the worst offenders when it comes to salt. White bread is particularly bad and, as we know, it has very low nutritional value. Many brown breads can also contain large amounts of salt, so the best thing would be to buy from a health-food shop or simply make your own.

2 **Cheese** is a preserved food, which basically means it contains high levels of salt (especially hard cheese such as Parmesan that takes longer to mature). To cut down on your cheese intake, try limiting the amount of cheese you eat by using it as an addition to salads or a food topping. The popular choice for many is cottage cheese, since it is deemed to be the healthy option. Where possible, opt for low-fat or fat-free versions, which tend to contain less salt. Mozzarella, ricotta and cream cheese are all good options.

Be aware of where the hidden salt lies.

 Crisps are not the healthiest thing you could be snacking on and they are very high in salt. It is possible to get reduced-salt versions, but if you are serious about losing weight crisps are best avoided.

 Pasta sauces that you buy in the supermarket are known to be another salt culprit. Obviously the quantity of salt added depends on the brand, but it would be much better to cook your own sauce from scratch. Use fresh tomatoes, basil, garlic and chillies to make a tasty and nutritious option.

 Bacon is one of the biggest sources of salt in many people's diet. Anyone who is worried about their blood pressure needs to eliminate it altogether as many brands contain 1g salt per rasher.

 Breakfast cereals: Many can be surprisingly high in salt. Try to eat porridge oats or reduced-salt muesli instead.

 Pizza is a popular treat for many, but be aware that takeaway pizzas and those bought from the supermarket can be full of salt. The only way to control what you eat is to make your own dough and sauce at home.

 Soy sauce is an obvious choice for making a simple stir-fry at home, but always go for the low fat option that tends to contain less salt as well.

 Olives soaked in brine: Olives are rich in antioxidants and vitamin E, meaning they are really good for you, but unfortunately the ones soaked in brine contain high levels of salt. Instead, go for varieties that are soaked in water. Even though the taste is slightly bitter, they are much healthier.

 Salted nuts are obviously extremely high in salt, so always choose unsalted versions.

One teaspoon of sugar contains 16kcal.

How to beat a sugar addiction

Are you a sugar addict? Can you go a day without it? Do you have a really sweet tooth? If the answer is 'yes', you are not on your own! As in the case of salt, there is sugar in many processed foods. Of course, we know that all cakes, pastries, sweets and chocolate contain plenty of the ingredient, but there are also many items that you wouldn't expect to contain sugar which actually do. For example, sugar can be found in jars of pasta sauce, ketchup, bread, cereals, juices and smoothies. And the problem with these products is it isn't always the natural kind. In an attempt to make their foods more enticing, manufacturers also sneak in refined sugar – and in many cases, they don't make this clear on the labels. This is what makes many of these products addictive and why many people find that they crave these foods all the time.

If this sounds familiar, there are steps you can take to try to overcome the cravings you feel. Unfortunately, losing weight and continuing to eat sugary food don't go together. It's time to cut out the everyday treats and get back to basics with natural and wholesome foods that should satisfy you without the consequences appearing on your tummy! One of the things I did was give up chocolate completely as this was the sugary snack I loved most. I just found it was easier to cut it out rather than be tempted! There is nothing to stop you treating yourself to something at the weekends, but do try to change your everyday habits if they include too much sugar otherwise you will be unlikely to lose weight in the way you hope to.

The other fact to be aware of is that eating too much sugar can put you at serious risk of developing type 2 diabetes. It's an increasing problem in today's society for the very reason that so much of what we eat contains large amounts of sugar.

More specifically, research has linked sugary soft drinks to the disease. Type 2 diabetes often goes undiagnosed for a long time because it doesn't always have obvious symptoms. The positive news is that it can be helped through diet and exercise.

Banishing the sugar

It's time to say 'no' to dessert and pass on the chocolate with your tea break. Here are some of my tips for cutting down on sugar:

 Clear out your cupboards of any foods containing refined sugar, as you don't want to be tempted every time you are hungry. Things like pasta sauces, tomato ketchup, peanut butter and tinned fruit are all culprits. It is the hidden sugars that we must be aware of.

 Avoid the aisle in the supermarket that you know is filled with the sugary items you love. It's the only way to eliminate temptation.

 Substitute sweet desserte with a piece of fruit: If dessert is your weakness, finish your evening meal with a piece of fruit to satisfy your sweet tooth. Why not try a baked apple or a poached pear?

 Try new foods! When we eat too much sugar our taste buds become affected and it can take a while to get used to real food again. Don't be afraid to experiment. Buy a new cookbook with healthy recipes and begin to enjoy flavours that you have been missing out on.

 Wean yourself off sugar in your tea and coffee: One teaspoon of sugar contains 16kcal. According to the American Heart Association, we should not be exceeding 100 calories of sugar per day. This is the equivalent of six teaspoons. The sugar that people add to coffee and tea can be extremely addictive, so that's a habit you need to break. If it means not buying sugar for a while, that's what you have to do. Alternatively, try making small adjustments each day or every week – cutting down from two teaspoons to one, say, in the beginning. This is a good way to adjust and I'm pretty sure you won't miss it once you make the change.

The truth about fast food

All around the world we are quickly becoming fast-food followers. Over the years we have seen a dramatic rise in the number of franchised fast-food outlets being opened. In fact, it's very hard to avoid them. What once started out as a novelty for children is quickly taking over our life. If we don't drive by one, we see advertisements on TV or in magazines to remind us of their ever-increasing presence. What does this mean for our health as a nation and how do we prevent people from making terrible food choices?

As already experienced by our North American counterparts, the effects of consuming too much fast food are starting to show in the UK. You only have to look around to see that the problem with weight and obesity is on the rise. There appears to be no 'stop' button. It's not enough to bury our heads in the sand in the hope that the problem will miraculously go away; we have to educate ourselves so we can make informed decisions in the future. I'm pretty sure that if you knew all the facts about what fast food contains you might reconsider paying regular visits to these restaurants. Apart from anything else, this type of food is very destructive for you in your bid to lose weight.

Extremely clever and catchy marketing campaigns mean that we are constantly aware of the latest specials at fast-food restaurants. Maybe it's a burger for £1 or 'Buy one portion of chips and get another free'. Well, if you're a fast-food lover this can be very tempting and probably hard to walk past. But the truth is that many of these places have begun to lull us into a false sense of security by making claims that their food has a level of nutritional value. It seems like a contradiction in terms. I find it hard to believe that there is anything nutritious about fast food. It comes down to the fact that most fast food is over-processed, which basically means that any goodness has been removed. Processed meat, processed cheese, processed bread, the list is endless. This is the type of food that is not only damaging to your weight loss, but also dangerous to your health. Apart from containing a huge amount of calories, fast food also contains additives, including MSG. It is literally designed to make you want more, making it highly addictive. Why else do you think people keep going back?

How to say 'no' to fast food
By eating this type of food regularly you are actually starving your body of the vitamins and minerals that it needs to work properly. The first thing you must do is figure out how you can eliminate fast food from your diet. Here are some tips:

- If fast food is something you crave after you've had a bad day, plan ahead. Instead of stopping off for a greasy burger and chips on the way home, plan a trip to the supermarket and pick up some fresh ingredients. Treat yourself to a home-cooked meal that you really enjoy.

- If you find that after a night out you tend to crave fast food, be prepared for that eventuality. Have something ready in the fridge that you can enjoy instead.

- If your excuse is that ordering fast food is quicker after a hectic day, start cooking extra with your evening meals and freezing a portion to have another day. This way, you won't be stuck when it comes to dinnertime and you'll be less lightly to grab something you shouldn't.

- If you are always tempted by the lure of additive-filled fast food, avoid the temptation. Walk a different route home from work or drive another way to make sure you are not confronted with the enemy!

- Why not cook your own healthy (and tastier) versions of fast food, such as homemade burgers or oven-baked chicken goujons in breadcrumbs?

- Stay focused. Keep thinking of the efforts you are making towards shedding the pounds and try not to lose sight of your goal. Making healthy choices isn't always easy when you're trying to fight the habit of a lifetime; however, fast food will never be the answer.

The truth about eating slowly

I'm always on the go, always rushing like most busy mums to the next meeting or to pick the kids up from school. Life is busy and I like it that way, but it can cause problems when it comes to losing weight. Years ago, when I found myself having a day that was non-stop, I used to grab food on the go. I'd stop at the nearest garage or coffee shop and I never chose the healthy option! I was in a rush and so I told myself that I needed fast food. It just seemed easier and we can all be guilty of that. The fast food that I usually picked up would be eaten very quickly and I probably didn't taste it properly. All it did was provide me with the sudden burst of energy I craved. Shortly afterwards, the crash would come and before long I'd find myself back to square one and starving again. Being stressed or under pressure certainly prevents us from thinking clearly.

No matter how busy life is, you have to eat. Digestion is part of that, so why not do it properly? In 1986, an initiative was developed in Italy called the Slow Food Movement. It was originally set up as an alternative to the fast-food and fast-life mentality that appeared to be taking over. Slow food is now active all over the world and it really has got people thinking about how they view food. The aim of the movement is to promote local food traditions and people's interest in the food they eat, where it comes from and how it tastes. It's all about getting back to basics and appreciating what we eat.

The good news, ladies, is that studies have shown that by eating slowly you will consume fewer calories. But how do you retrain your brain to do this? Well, one of the first things you have to do is to learn to enjoy the art of eating.

Slow down, what's the sense in rushing?
Whatever is happening in your day, take time out to slow down the pace and really enjoy your food. Taste what you're eating and take in the flavours. How many of us grab a bite to eat too quickly? Eating slowly means you are in the moment and not worrying or stressing about what you have to do next. If you

Studies have shown that by eating slowly you will consume fewer calories.

get into a routine of doing this, not only will you learn to appreciate the food but also you will find that your appetite is reduced.

This might sound silly, but very often when people are really hungry they forget to chew. Chewing both breaks down the food and sends a message to the digestive organs to prepare for food. The digestion process starts in your mouth and chewing properly allows for easier digestion. In other words, the more slowly you eat, the more able you are to metabolise your food. If you eat without chewing, the food in your mouth becomes harder for your body to break down. Eating too much food too quickly could cause indigestion. That feeling of being so full you feel uncomfortable isn't good for you. It's time to knock it on the head and learn to chew your food properly.

Drinking at mealtimes

Without wishing to sound like a broken record, I can't stress enough that the better the food you eat, the better it is for your digestion. Our body wasn't built to digest additives and overprocessed foods. Set time aside for your meals every day and discover the benefits of eating slowly.

Research has shown that drinking cold drinks with food may not be the best thing for the digestive system. Cold drinks slow down the digestive process so the food can't break down properly, meaning it's harder for your body to extract the energy and nutrients it needs. Now I know you may not want to drink tea with your stir-fry or salad, but a good tip is to retrain yourself to drink water before your meal and limit yourself to taking just small sips of water while you are eating. Another good practice is to drink a mug of hot water with freshly squeezed lemon or lime juice in it first thing in the morning, which will cleanse your stomach and stimulate the digestion ready for the day ahead.

Learning from other cultures

According to the British Heart Foundation, heart and circulatory diseases cause more than a quarter of all deaths in the UK each year. The figure is the same in the US. And in Australia, the Heart Foundation claims that cardiovascular disease is the leading cause of death. It is said to kill one Australian every 12 minutes. These figures are shocking, and yet the facts aren't the same everywhere in the world. Statistics have shown that the Italians, for example, are far less likely to die from cancer and heart problems than their British and Irish counterparts. What is their secret? And is there something we can learn from other cultures?

The Italian way

The Italian culture of eating *al fresco*, around a big table and involving all the family, is such a fantastic way of life. There is a social aspect to Italians' meal times – they are often found sitting for hours over a lovingly prepared meal, or even a simple cup of coffee. Now, granted, they do enjoy a slightly better climate than us. But the thing I admire is how their focus is always on spending time together, not on rushing their food or eating on the go. Eating in front of the television just wouldn't be considered the norm for them. It is their belief that food is something that brings people together – hence time and energy go into the whole cooking process. Wholefoods and market-bought ingredients, coupled with sensible portions, are what keep the Italians healthy and happy. It's for these very reasons that they have one of the lowest obesity rates in the world.

So what makes the Italian diet so special? Italians are well known for their coffee and usually start their day with a strong cup accompanied by a large glass of water. Lunch and dinner are traditionally split into a 'first' and 'second' plate. The first plate usually consists of pasta with a freshly made tomato or vegetable sauce. The portion of pasta is small and the sauce rarely involves cream. The second part of the meal is generally either fish or chicken. They don't eat red meat very often. This combination means that they are getting a meal that is equally balanced between carbohydrates and protein. They take breaks between courses, meaning a dinner can last for many hours. This is where they are getting it so right, allowing plenty of time to digest the food and enjoy the experience of eating.

So is it possible to adopt the Italian way of eating? When cooking they only use olive oil, and they use it sparingly. And, again, when they do use salt they don't add too much. They prefer to flavour food with garlic, black pepper and herbs. When it comes to salad dressings, they are much more likely to drizzle on a dash of balsamic vinegar and olive oil – they believe that you need only a small amount. They don't slather mayonnaise over everything like we tend to. As you can see, their secret is simple: everything in its pure form and in modest amounts.

The Chinese secret

The Chinese food I'm referring to here is not the kind you order from your local Chinese restaurant on a Saturday night. That version has been modified to suit Western tastes, which have become accustomed to overprocessed and fatty foods. I'm talking about the sort of food that people enjoy at home in China. So what is the Chinese secret?

One of the things you will notice when you go into any Chinese restaurant is how customers eat out of small bowls. They are very strict on portion control. When you think about it logically, the size of your plate definitely impacts on the amount of food you eat. I've already talked about the importance of eating slowly and how it triggers your digestion if you chew your food carefully. Well, one of the things the Chinese are known for are their chopsticks! Eating quickly simply isn't possible when you use chopsticks.

Like Italians, most Chinese people favour freshly cooked food. Plus, in China, vegetables are considered as integral to the meal as meat. Root vegetables, in particular, are especially important – not only are they rich in fibre, but also they are full of health benefits. Another very healthy part of the Chinese diet is tea – both green and herbal. They don't use milk or cream; the tea they drink is rich in antioxidants. Green and herbal teas are great for aiding the digestion and are known to boost the metabolism naturally. Another benefit is that tea helps to alleviate hunger – so the next time you feel like snacking, you know what to reach for!

When it comes to being fit, the Chinese are fans of what is known as restorative exercise, which is all about balance, vitality and flexibility. T'ai chi is often practised after a meal in order to maintain an active metabolism. It is a low-impact, slow-motion form of exercise that is often described as 'meditation in motion'. In so many ways the Chinese have struck a positively healthy balance between what they eat and their lifestyle.

Beware the Chinese takeaway!

If you are watching your weight and think it's safe to ring up for a Chinese takeaway on a Saturday night, think again. A recent survey carried out by Safefood (a government body) in Ireland revealed shocking results in relation to the average Chinese takeaway. A dinner serving for one, which typically includes vegetable spring rolls, sweet-and-sour chicken and egg-fried rice, contains 2,184 calories. This accounts for about 109 per cent of your recommended daily calorie intake. It's the equivalent of nine Mars bars or 66 chicken nuggets in one sitting! It also contains 70g fat and 10g salt. Next time, will you still tempted to pick up the phone? I hope not.

Chapter seven

The benefits
OF EATING WELL

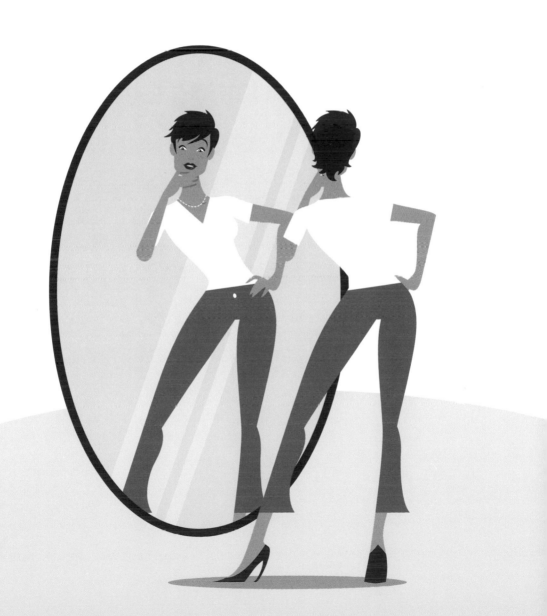

Sooner or later bad eating habits will catch up with you.

Feeding our skin, hair and nails

You can own every make-up and haircare product in the world, which of course will help you look fabulous, but the real answer to healthy skin, strong nails and gorgeous locks has so much to do with the foods we eat.

Do you really think that a greasy burger and chips could have a positive impact on your skin? It comes down to one simple fact, and it's nothing new: you are what you eat. If you have been living on an unhealthy diet and believe you are getting away with it, rest assured that your immunity won't last forever! Sooner or later bad eating habits will catch up with you. Switching to a healthy diet to lose weight can also benefit how you look in so many ways. What you eat really does impact your appearance.

Drinking water is a must for healthy-looking skin. Drinking it regularly helps keep you hydrated, which is really important if you find that you suffer from dry skin patches. Sometimes it's hard to get into a routine of sipping water during the day, so if this is an issue try switching to green tea instead. This can be really effective because of the antioxidants it contains, which are great for the skin. Remember that most fruit and vegetables have a high water content – opt for melon, cucumbers, peppers and oranges to keep your skin hydrated. Oranges, in particular, are packed full of vitamin C, which can help to strengthen the skin. Make sure you stock up on carrots, too, as they are great for keeping the skin clear and they are full of vitamin A. Flax seeds, which contain omega-3 fatty acids, are said to be helpful when it comes to treating skin conditions such as eczema. If you're not sure how to include them in your diet, try scattering them over your porridge in the morning or sprinkling some over salad or soup during the day. Also make sure you get your fill of almonds, which are high in vitamin E, something we all need in the fight against sun damage.

Healthy hair is something that we women always strive for. We spend so much on treatments and serum and they often cost a small fortune. So wouldn't it be nice to think that if we ate the right foods we could have beautiful hair and more money in our wallet? Vitamin D is a must to keep your hair shiny and vibrant, and fish such as salmon or mackerel are all good sources, as are avocados. Eggs contain the B vitamin biotin, which is great for stimulating hair growth. Olive oil is good for giving hair shine, so make sure you get some every day. To give hair strength, try to include plenty of iron in your diet – beef, peanuts and lentils are all good sources. Zinc, too, is helpful in preventing hair loss – find it in shellfish, beef, lamb and peanuts.

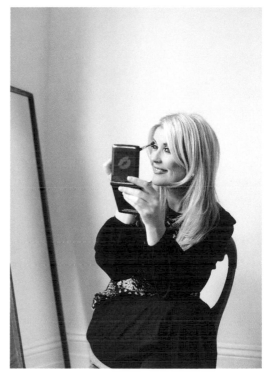

Many people wonder why their nails are brittle and never grow. Again it all comes down to feeding yourself well in order to see the results on the outside. All the B vitamins are useful for nail growth and these can be found in eggs, yogurt, tomatoes, carrots and raspberries. We were told when we were younger that our bones needed calcium. This is equally true for our nails, so try to include some dairy produce in your diet. Zinc and vitamin C are also great for maintaining strong nails.

Foods to keep you looking younger

Hold your hands up high, ladies: how many of you are constantly being lured into buying the latest anti-wrinkle cream or anti-ageing serum? Throughout our lifetime we spend a small fortune on cosmetics and skincare products in an

Feed yourself well in order to see the results on the outside.

attempt to fight the signs of ageing and grow old gracefully. But what we often overlook is the fact that our appearance and how we age are not down to the cream we apply on our skin. Of course, some products are great and contain ingredients that work for us. But staying youthful on the outside has so much more to do with our lifestyle and diet. Think of someone you know who has aged well. Chances are they take care of their body from the inside out. It's all about feeding ourselves with the right ingredients in order for the results to show on our face and body. Yes, it's as simple as that – the secret to younger-looking skin could be sitting in your fridge drawer!

Fruit and vegetables

Start the day in the best possible way with citrus fruits such as oranges, lemons or grapefruits. Not only are these packed with vitamin C, which we know is great for our immune system, but they are a secret to younger-looking skin too. Vitamin C is required to help cleanse your skin and give it a healthy glow, which we all want. It is also responsible for building collagen, which is essential for keeping the skin radiant and fresh. While citrus fruits are well-known sources of vitamin C, you can also get your daily intake from sweet peppers, blackcurrants or tomatoes. And the good thing about tomatoes is that, as well as containing lots of vitamin C, they are also rich in antioxidants, which are essential in helping to protect our skin from sun damage. We have all heard in the last few years about 'superfoods' and on that list are blueberries. These are really rich in antioxidants, which help to protect your skin from premature ageing. A great way to eat them is on top of your porridge or cereal in the morning.

Most people know that vitamin E is essential for healthy, young-looking skin and this is found in a wide variety of vegetables – in particular, avocados, tomatoes, spinach and broccoli. Vitamin E is also found in walnuts, almonds, sunflower seeds and pine nuts, to name but a few, so there are plenty of options for your everyday diet.

The secret to younger-looking skin could be sitting in your fridge drawer!

Potatoes

When it comes to potatoes, forget the original spud and opt for the sweet version. This is a much better choice for a healthy diet and it also contains beta-carotene, which is known to help our skin stay smoother since it balances the pH. This is especially important during the cold winter months when the weather can really play havoc with our skin, leaving it feeling rough and dried out.

Fish

If you are looking for the perfect food, you won't go wrong with a piece of salmon. This fish is rich in omega-3, which is said to be great for fighting wrinkles. More than ever we are being advised that a diet rich in fish is really beneficial for us. If fish just isn't for you, a good alternative would be to start taking a fish-oil supplement every day.

Wholegrains

If you decide to give up one thing today, make sure you wave goodbye to refined grains and switch to the whole versions. White foods such as bread, pasta and rice cause the collagen in our skin to become inflamed, which is one of the things that causes wrinkles. Wholegrain versions, on the other hand, are rich in antioxidants and also contain fibre, which is essential for younger-looking skin.

Salt and sugar

Cutting back on the amount of salt you use is another step in the right direction. So many processed foods contain large amounts of salt that the only way you can be sure of reducing your intake is to cook food yourself. We all need a certain amount of salt, but too much in your diet can leave your skin looking bloated and tired. Similarly, sugary foods have a negative effect on the skin. This is yet another reason to eliminate the cakes, pastries and sugary drinks from your diet! They could be the cause if your skin is dull and lacking in vitality. It's time to lose the salt and sugar if you long for vibrant and bright-looking skin.

Dark chocolate

Yes, you read that right! Cocoa beans are rich in antioxidants, which means they are actually good for you, in moderation of course. Dark chocolate contains a much higher cocoa content than the milk version and therefore is always the one to go for. The antioxidants that it contains are good for protecting your heart against disease and ageing, while the flavonoids help blood flow to the skin and improve hydration. Isn't that the best news ever?

Nothing tastes as good as sexy feels!

Foods to boost your sex drive

In 1996 a survey was carried out in America which showed that the average American was having sex 138 times a year. Fast-forward to 2007 and figures showed the average American was having sex only 85 times a year. So why have the numbers dropped and what has changed?

Experts maintain that these figures clearly portray the growing problem people are having with their weight and how it is affecting their confidence and performance in the bedroom. Nutritionists say that there is a definite link between our libido and what we eat. In order to have a healthy sex life, it stands to reason that you need to have a healthy body. So what changes can we make to our food plan if we are experiencing problems in this area?

If you want to be sure that you will be eating a libido-enhancing meal, the best thing you can do is learn to cook in the comfort of your own home. That way, you have total control over what goes in the pot! Forget the traditional idea that you have in your head of a rich meal in a fancy restaurant. There is nothing romantic about feeling bloated. Also, if you really want to help yourself, cut back on the alcohol. It might boost your confidence, but the chemicals it contains will have the opposite effect on your sex drive. Try to limit yourself to about two drinks. As Shakespeare once said, 'It provokes the desire but it takes away the performance'!

In terms of your diet, there are plenty of things you can eat to get your evening off to a good start. Begin your meal with some asparagus. It could be grilled, roasted or steamed. The great thing about asparagus is that it's rich in vitamin E (known as the 'sex vitamin'!), which is said to stimulate the production of sex hormones. Another good starter is avocado, which is rich in vitamin B6 and folic acid, which help provide the body with more sexual energy.

Moving on to the main course, here it's all about getting your blood moving, and the best thing to serve up if you want to boost your sex drive is fish – in particular, oily fish such as salmon or mackerel, which are both rich in omega-3 fatty acids. Try to cook them with garlic, if that won't put your partner off, as this is meant to improve your blood circulation. Serve with green leafy vegetables, which are packed with iron to give you energy, and plenty of basil to boost your fertility and increase circulation – basil is also thought to arouse males and is good for stimulating the sex drive, so you can't go far wrong with this one.

Instead of a rich sugary dessert, which might sound delicious but will leave you feeling bloated and lethargic, try always to opt for something that is going to compliment your meal. Bananas are full of potassium and a good source of B vitamins. This means they will provide you with lots of much-needed energy! If you're not a banana lover, why not opt for strawberries dipped in dark chocolate instead. Strawberries are a rich source of folic acid, while dark chocolate contains antioxidants to help improve blood-vessel function, which means they are both great for your libido.

Of course, these are all examples of specific foods that could boost your libido if you are having a romantic night in. However, as I have stressed before, the key to being healthy is all about making lifestyle changes, including changing how you cook your food. Remember that all foods containing large amounts of saturated fat (see page 79) are bad for you, and they are also the worst foods you could eat for your sex drive. The message is clear: if you want to get things moving in the bedroom, you have to make changes in the kitchen too!

To get things moving in the bedroom, make changes in the kitchen too!

> *Choose something that you will enjoy or have always wanted to try.*

Love life? Love to live longer?

We have always been well informed about the things in life that are supposedly meant to keep us looking and feeling younger – lotions, potions, water, fruit and vegetables, plenty of sleep, lots of exercise… the list goes on and on! However, while these are all great ways to stay healthy and in shape, there are other influences in our life that could play a part. I'm definitely a big believer in living life to the full because we only get one shot at it. I like to think that, for the most part, I have made the most of any opportunities that have come my way. I have always done what I can to challenge myself and have been open to try new things. Losing weight did change many things for me, but at the very top of that list would be discovering the importance of living life to the full. Why wouldn't I? I have my family, health and happiness.

Lisa's tips for living life to the full

Aside from all the things you are already doing to keep the weight off, what else can you do to improve your life and hopefully live longer? The good news is that there are lots of options. Here are my top seven tips:

 Take up a new hobby or learn a new skill: It's all about getting your brain active and pushing yourself in as many ways as you can. As we get older it's even more important to keep the mind active. It helps to stimulate our brain and allows it to function better. Choose something that you will enjoy or have always wanted to try. This will ensure that you get the most out of whatever it is.

 Have more sex! Being intimate with your partner is good for your health and is well known to keep stress levels at bay. People who enjoy an active sex life are said to get a much better night's sleep and are generally happier. You heard it here first: what a fun way to add extra years to your life!

Take plenty of tea breaks: Tea offers a number of benefits. It has an amazing ability to provide a source of comfort for people when they need it. In many cases, a cup of tea has even been known to solve problems! Tea is also rich in antioxidants, which we need to keep us healthy.

 Get a pet: As well as giving you lots of love and attention, a pet is a brilliant way of encouraging you to get outdoors and become more active. Having a pet gives you another focus, which can be very important at certain stages in life.

 Develop meaningful relationships: Getting on well with people and developing special bonds is said to make us happy. Happier people are generally healthier and they have a more positive outlook on life – research even suggests that optimistic people tend to outlive those who are pessimistic.

 Laugh as much as you can: The old saying 'Laughter is the best medicine' is so true. A good dose of laughter is great for the soul and can also be a great stress reliever.

Get married! Research has shown that married people are, for the most part, happier than those who are unmarried. However crazy it may sound, divorced and single people have an increased risk of dying at an earlier age.

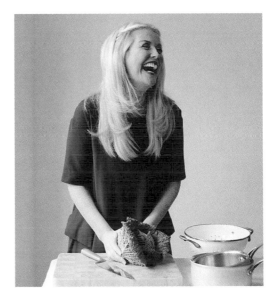

Chapter eight

Strategies TO KEEP YOU ON TRACK

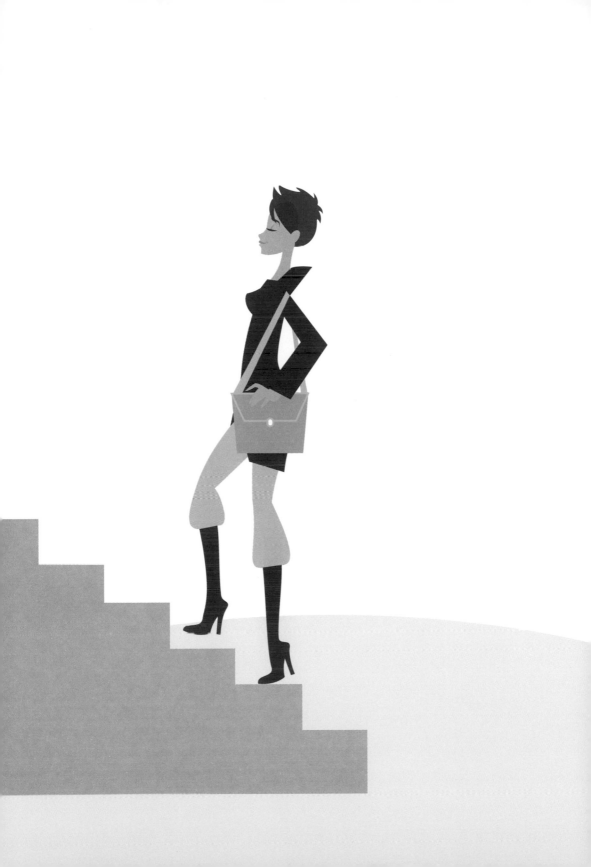

Take small steps to begin with and persevere.

However firm your resolve, there will inevitably be times when you deviate from your diet, so what follows are some tips and strategies that have helped me.

Developing good habits

There is often the misconception that making a lifestyle change is all about food and exercise. This couldn't be further from the truth. There are so many other factors that come into play. These tips might sound simple but putting them into practice could be harder than you think. Take small steps to begin with and persevere. If it helps, try writing out this list and putting it on the front of the fridge to keep you focused.

Skipping meals is one of the worst things you can do and, contrary to what you might believe, it does not help you to lose weight. What happens is that your metabolism rate slows down as your body goes into what is known as 'starvation mode'. In order to preserve itself the body then goes on to burn muscle and the next time you eat any excess calories will be stored as fat. Whenever you think that missing lunch is going to help your weight loss, remember the science behind it.

- **Start your day with a healthy breakfast:** There is truth in the saying that breakfast is the most important meal of the day. It sets you up for what's ahead and helps provide you with the energy you need to kickstart the day. Try to avoid cereals that are high in sugar and salt. Usually wholegrain and bran-based ones are a better option. A good breakfast means you are less likely to feel a mid-morning slump, which often causes people to crave sugar. For more healthy breakfast ideas, see page 130.

- **Drink eight glasses of water every day:** Carrying a bottle of water in your bag will help you cut back on fizzy drinks, tea and coffee, all of which can be laden with sugar and very addictive. Drinking water before you eat means you won't feel as hungry, plus it's also a great way to make sure you stay hydrated and avoid feeling drained and unenergised.

- **Cook your meals from scratch:** If you can prepare your food from scratch at home, do so. That way you have total control over what you are eating. Cooking for yourself can be relaxing, so try not to see it as a chore.

- **Reduce your portion size:** It's quite straightforward when you think about it. If you consume more calories than you burn, you will put on weight because your body stores them up as fat. One of the easiest ways to work on portion control is to use a smaller plate. If someone else serves you, don't feel obliged to eat everything on your plate. You should eat until you feel full or satisfied.

- **Use herbs and spices to flavour food:** As lovely as dressings and sauces taste, they are usually heavy on calories as well as your stomach! Sauces were one of the things that definitely contributed to my weight gain. Herbs and spices provide lots of flavour without causing you to pile on the pounds.

- **Ditch the deep-fat fryer:** Frying automatically adds calories to your food. Instead try grilling, roasting, poaching or boiling food. These are much better methods and ensure that your food retains the nutrients that you need for a healthy diet.

- **Limit your alcohol intake:** Bad news, ladies – alcohol is not great for weight loss. It contains empty calories and also affects your ability to burn fat. Try to cut back if you can. That way, the next time you have a glass it will taste even better!

- **Get a good night's sleep:** The lack of a good night's sleep can affect our thinking. When we don't sleep well, we don't function well – ideally you need eight hours every night, or as close to this as possible. Think about it in terms of looking after your body and wellbeing. Being tired can often lead you to eat the wrong type of food. This is especially true when you are new mum. I remember having tea and toast at four in the morning and looking forward to it!

- **Try not to stress:** When life is busy it is easy to feel the weight of the world on your shoulders. Unfortunately for many of us stress can lead to an increase in appetite, which in turn can lead to weight gain. Try to find a way of relaxing when you feel as if things are getting on top of you. Going for a walk and breathing some fresh air can be a great way of clearing your head.

- **Persevere:** A lot of these tips took me months to get my head around. It was like retraining my brain. I had to learn to fight the cravings, fill myself with the right foods and allow the fact that I felt better to provide me with proof that my new lifestyle was working. Remember, it won't all happen at once.

Keeping a food journal

The idea of writing down what you eat every day can be daunting because it means facing up to the truth about your diet. When it's written down you have to face up to reality. An extra biscuit or two here, the odd packet of sneaky crisps that you'd forgotten about! When it's all written down, it is much harder to ignore. Keeping a food journal is a good lesson in making us aware of our eating habits and may be something that actively encourages change. I kept a journal for four months when I was starting out on my battle to lose weight and I learned a lot about food during that time. It worked for me because I got to see what I was really eating and it allowed me to make changes accordingly. It's not something

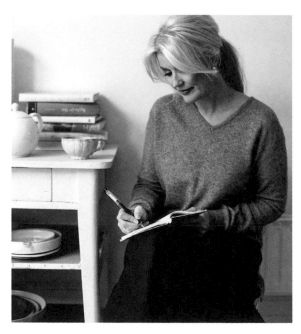

I want you to become obsessive over, but it is worth doing for a short period of time. In my case, it helped me to focus on where I needed more variety in my diet and also where I needed to cut back. In particular, it is a good way of establishing whether you are eating a balanced diet that is rich in protein, minerals, vitamins, carbohydrates and fat (see pages 74–95).

Finding a diet that works for you

You will learn new things as you set out on this journey and discovering new foods is a great part of that. Enjoying your meals every day and eating food that you like will make the transition that little bit easier. It might surprise you to discover that good food actually tastes good! My daily diet now is far removed from what I previously ate, and yet I can honestly say I don't miss a thing and wouldn't want to go back to the way things were. I am also proud of the fact that my children and husband eat healthily now, because I do, and I feel a strong sense of responsibility towards them.

This is an example of the daily regime that works for me (for sample recipes, see pages 128–159):

My daily regime

7am: Cup of coffee and a wholegrain biscuit. (I try to avoid eating breakfast immediately I get up.)

10am: Breakfast: For me, this is the most important meal of the day, so I try to have something substantial that will see me through to lunch, such as poached eggs on toast, or a bowl of porridge with fresh fruit. I cut out bread completely Monday to Friday.

1pm: Lunch: If I'm at home I have salad for lunch or homemade soup. Otherwise I take a packed lunch so I'm less tempted by unhealthy choices.

3pm: I like to have a cup of refreshing green tea. If I'm feeling a little hungry I'll snack on raw vegetables or a small granola bar. If I'm out, I always go prepared with a little bag of tricks!

6pm: If I'm hungry around this time I'll just have some water and a handful of nuts or dried fruit. It's so important not to spoil your main meal.

7pm: At home during the week, I love doing chicken or beef stir-fries. They are quick and easy but also nutritious. If I'm out for dinner, I'll usually opt for the fish and make sure to ask for any sauces to be served on the side.

You can't eat foods you enjoy and it seems like the end of the world!

Maintaining a healthy attitude towards food

One of the most dominant feelings you may have when you start to change your diet and lifestyle is that you are being deprived – suddenly you can't eat a whole list of foods you enjoy and, quite frankly, it seems like the end of the world! This is something that many women can relate to. They start their diet on a Monday and spend the day consumed by thoughts of foods they must avoid. By the end of the day they have tortured themselves to the point where the diet is forgotten and they have convinced themselves that some nice food will make them feel better. This is not a cycle I want you to repeat. What you need to get you through this journey is a healthy attitude towards food and that means focusing your energy on all the foods you are going to try, not the ones you must eat less of.

Food shopping can be one of the biggest tests for anyone trying to stick to a healthy diet. So I recommend three things to ensure the items in your trolley don't go off message.

Supermarket tips

- **Do not do your weekly shop when you are hungry:** If you do, you're almost guaranteed to buy all the things you shouldn't. Eat before you leave so that you are in the right frame of mind and therefore less likely to be distracted.

- **Make a list:** If it's written out you will be focused on what you have to buy, not what you need to avoid. It's about taking control. Plan your menus for the week ahead using recipes from this book and also start experimenting with your own.

- **Read the labels:** That old saying, 'Knowledge is power', comes into play here. If you really want to know what you are eating, read the labels attached to the food you are buying. Too often we are more interested in getting value for money than making healthier choices.

Changing your eating habits for good

It's just as easy to eat good food as it is bad. Each and every one of us has a different attitude towards food. Some people claim to be overeaters and just can't help themselves. Others can go for long periods without so much as a bite of food passing their lips. Whatever your pattern has been up to this point, it's time to change your approach to food, start making the right choices and really develop healthy eating habits. Change will come if you are willing to try.

1. Emotional eating

Our emotions have a massive effect on the way we eat. For some people, the first thing they do when they are going through a tough time is to reach for the nearest carbohydrate. For others, food is the furthest thing from their mind. In order to lose weight you have to be willing to explore the foods you eat and understand why you eat them. What is the trigger that makes you crave the wrong foods and how can you overcome it?

One of the standout moments for me took place at Barcelona airport a few years back. I had accompanied my husband on a business trip – there were about 50 people in the group – and we had had a great time. However, on the way back, the security guard asked me to remove my shoes at the airport. This was fine. She then asked me to remove my coat. This was not fine. Underneath I knew my trouser zip wouldn't close and I could feel my large tummy hanging out over the top. Immediately I panicked, felt my face go red and very reluctantly took off the coat. At that moment it felt like everything stopped. My heart sank and I imagined everyone was staring at me. It was pretty soul destroying to say the least. I pulled myself together, went to the bathroom and called my mum. Being the kind and wonderful woman that my mum is she said, 'Lisa, you're beautiful! Go and have a nice cup of tea and a muffin'. Sometimes food is associated with providing comfort and this is a perfect example. As much as I love my mum, I think a muffin was the last thing I actually needed back then.

It's just as easy to eat good food as it is bad.

If you can train yourself to think past the food, you should feel less tempted by it.

Like it or not, emotional eating has the power to damage the steps you are taking towards your weight loss. Consciously or unconsciously food can provide comfort during stressful times, but in many cases it can also lead to overeating. That overeating can then become part of a cycle. If you associate stress or being upset with food, it is bound to be your first port of call. However, if you can train yourself to think past the food, you should feel less tempted by it. If you want to break the cycle, you need to find an alternative way to comfort yourself, such as having a bath, reading a book or going for a walk. I often find in these situations that any distraction at all is the best way to overcome temptation – I sit down and get cosy in front of the TV or do my to-do list for the next day. It's all about finding a distraction that works for you.

2. Junk-food cravings

When I started losing weight the biggest change I made was in the type of food I ate. I went from eating a calorie- and sugar-laden diet to making largely healthy choices. I was so used to eating badly that my body wasn't sure what was happening! Honestly, I thought I would crack up and I did falter on a number of occasions.

The biggest problem with junk food is it's addictive: the more you eat, the more you want to eat – you find your body literally calling out for sugar and carbs. However, the lousy way we feel after eating junk food is worth remembering. One of the steps I took to overcome my junk-food cravings was to keep a food diary and write down how I felt each time I ate junk – the words 'bloated', 'lacking in energy', 'guilty' and 'unhealthy' spring to mind! Writing down how you feel is a great way of reminding yourself next time you feel tempted. Here are some more tips to keep you motivated and help keep those cravings at bay:

- Always have a bottle of water handy – it's the best way to overcome cravings. Take a drink and see how you feel. Often when we think we're hungry, we're actually just dehydrated.
- Carry healthy snacks such as nuts or fruit with you at all times – these are

especially useful during the mid-morning slump when you often crave a bar of chocolate.

- Clear out your cupboards, fridge and freezer. Have a look through what you keep on the shelves. Be honest with yourself about how much of it is actually good for you. I'm not saying throw away absolutely everything, but if your cupboards are filled with nothing but treats you have no choice but to get rid of them! That is temptation staring you in the face.

3. Hangover cravings

That feeling of waking up with a fuzzy head and a dry mouth after a night of too much wine is very hard to forget. As we get older and our body slows down, we tend to feel the effects of a night out more than ever. It's a harsh, but very true, reality. If you are one of the lucky ones who doesn't suffer after overindulging, count your blessings, because for many of us it can be tough. Basically, we require a truckload of tea and sympathy! As lovely as a nice cup of tea is when you wake up with a blinding hangover, tea just doesn't cut the mustard. Ladies, let's lay our cards on the table. When we are feeling slightly delicate we want carbs and sugar. All the promises that we have made to ourselves soon become forgotten as our body calls out for something greasy and satisfying. We ignore our commitment to wholesome, nutritious foods because the hangover quite simply has a mind of its own. If you have been there and worn the t-shirt on more than one occasion, it might interest you to know that you can still have your favourite cures, but you just need to make some adjustments. So what do you do when you're trying to change your lifestyle, but your hangover says otherwise? You have to eat, but it must be a sensible choice that will still satisfy how you are feeling. Here are my top tips for surviving a hangover:

1 I have found something that works for me and it still tastes good. I eat poached eggs with homemade brown bread, accompanied by grilled tomatoes and water with grenadine. Ignore the sausage rolls and give this a go!

2 Forget the fry-up and get grilling. Grilling is a much healthier option and it means you can still enjoy your bacon. Make sure that you trim the fat from the bacon before you cook it. Have with a boiled or poached egg, which is rich in calcium and iron as well as being low in saturated fat. You could also have some baked beans if you like. This combination is perfect for keeping your diet healthy, but it will still hit the spot!

3 Another option would be to have some breakfast cereal. Any of the cereals that are high in fibre are what you need. If your stomach can handle it, drink some freshly squeezed fruit juice or a smoothie as well. These will provide you with a vitamin boost and they contain natural sugars to help with your hangover.

4 Have a hug! It might sound funny, but when you are feeling hungover and miserable, cuddles can help. It has been proved that having physical contact with another person can release a happy hormone. A hug won't take away how bad you feel, but it could ease the pain a little.

5 Get out and feel the air in your lungs. Sitting indoors and lazing on the couch all day will not make your hangover disappear. It just allows you to wallow in the guilt you feel from overindulging. Put your tracksuit on and go for a walk. Exercise is great for clearing your head and it also helps to increase circulation.

6 Drink water like there is no tomorrow! You know at this stage in your life that alcohol leaves you so dehydrated you feel like a camel that hasn't had water for days. So the next day, even if you are craving fizzy drinks, you must force yourself to drink water. If you find it hard, add grenadine, as I suggested in point one above. It gives it a slightly sweet taste and makes it easier to drink.

Coping with temptation

Sometimes it's hard to avoid temptation – it seems to be everywhere! You go to the shop to pick up a bottle of water and hundreds of glossy, shiny chocolate bars stare out at you lovingly. It's as if they are willing you to buy them. Or, in the coffee shop, the person behind the counter asks if you'd like something sweet to go with your Americano. Meanwhile, the muffins, chocolates and pastries are almost jumping from the shelves. Are you strong enough to walk away with your head held high, safe in the knowledge you have made the right decision? Some days it's easy to be strong and on others it feels like the most horrible test of willpower you've ever faced. This is perfectly normal, in case you were wondering. It's a battle many of us face on a regular basis, although the reasons why we overindulge differ from person to person. For some individuals, overindulging is an emotional response to a bad day – we are, literally, seeking comfort in food. For others, overindulging is the reward for a good day – we think we have earned the right to a treat. Remember that eating badly is not a reward. Whatever the cause of your overindulgence, here are some simple steps you can take both to rectify the situation and avoid it happening too often.

- **Accept that there will always be temptation:** We live in a world where advertising campaigns make food seem very appealing. At home, TV ads inform us about every kind of food imaginable. In our cars, we are bombarded with the same thing on the radio. In the course of our day, we pass billboards, posters, sweet shops, fast food restaurants and bakeries. This is life and it's not something we can avoid. All it means is that it's up to us to take charge of our life and not constantly give in to temptation. Think about the last time you overindulged. Did you feel good afterwards? Was it satisfying? Chances are that you felt sickly, uncomfortable, bloated and miserable. But it's a vicious circle and many of us repeat the process time after time. You have to stop letting food consume your thoughts and find a way of breaking bad habits.

- **It's not the end of the world if you've overindulged:** Look at it this way – tomorrow is another day, another chance to make amends. Go for a walk and clear your head. Often when we overeat we don't digest our food properly, which causes us to feel out-of-sorts. Walking is a great way to get your body moving again and it can also aid digestion. Make a plan for the next day that will include feeding your body with good foods – lean protein and fibre are

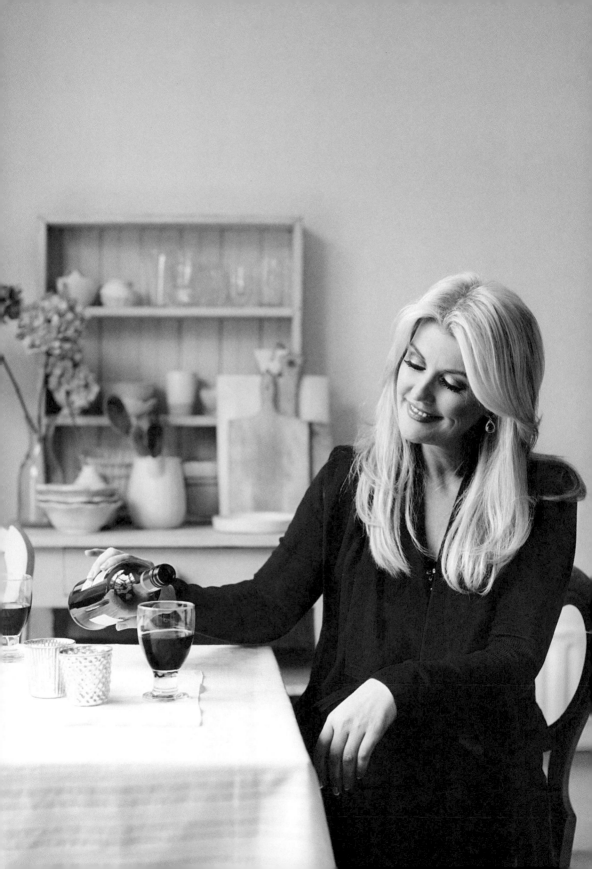

what you need if you have been overindulging in sugary and processed foods. Another tip is to drink herbal tea as it contains antioxidants and is great for cleansing your body.

- **Be prepared for the temptations that lie ahead:** Have your day mapped out in advance and have your food ready so that you won't be tempted by bad choices. Don't put yourself in situations where you will be confronted by the wrong foods. Out of sight is out of mind. Empty your shelves and fridge/ freezer now if you haven't already done so.

- **Listen to your body:** This is what people forget when they eat too much. You need to learn to recognise when you are truly hungry. Eating out of boredom is pointless, but many of us do it. Really ask yourself what your body needs and then satisfy that need in the best way you possibly can with healthy foods. In the same way, become aware of when you are actually full. Being full is not a feeling that makes you feel unwell; it's about recognising when you have had enough to eat. Eating is all about being in tune with your body and what it actually needs. Looking after your body means feeding your physical self and, in order to do this, you need to eat well. Right now, as I am writing this book, I feel cold. It's windy and miserable outside, but I'm having homemade soup instead of tea and biscuits. You will feel better if you give your body the vitamins and minerals it needs to be healthy. Keep this in mind each time you feel tempted to overindulge. Your body deserves only the best.

Dealing with obsessive thoughts

Apparently the average man thinks about sex once every hour of the day. Well, I am inclined to believe that one of the things that dominates many women's thoughts is weight loss! Whether it's food shopping with so many low fat options in the supermarket or a weight-loss programme on TV, dieting does seem to be everywhere. Do you wake up in the morning thinking about food and find you are still having those same thoughts when you go to bed at night? While a desire to be healthy, both in body and mind, is perfectly normal, an obsessive approach really isn't.

One of the most damaging consequences of having obsessive thoughts when we are trying to lose weight is that we often end up focusing on all the wrong things – namely, the foods we shouldn't be eating. It's very frustrating

You only have one body... take care of it.

because often our obsessive thoughts have a negative effect. If you spend your day fixated on what you are not supposed to have, the chances are you will find yourself seeking out the nearest sugary or fatty food no matter what it takes. You can't help it; your obsession has literally taken control. Here are some ways to take your attention away from the wrong food and help you to stay positive:

 Shift your focus: Yes, you have to make changes to your diet and your eating habits in general, but it is not the end of the world! What you need to concentrate on are all the healthy foods you are about to enjoy, maybe for the first time. Your new lifestyle means new recipes, enjoying new flavours and also being a bit more adventurous. Don't view this as something negative. Good food is good for you. It makes you feel better in every way. Try to change the way you view this and you are halfway there.

 See it as a lifestyle choice and reap the benefits: Leading a healthier lifestyle will not only help you to lose weight, but also it will make you feel better about yourself. Many things changed in my life when I lost weight and they were all for the best. Try it and you'll see!

 Plan your mealtimes and have snacks with you for during the day: This way, you know exactly what you are going to eat and when. If there is a definite structure to your day, it should help to eliminate those obsessive thoughts. They creep in when you have time on your hands, so being prepared is the only way to avoid this.

4 **Find an outlet:** If you continually obsess about food, you have to find something to do or somewhere to go when you feel these thoughts taking over. Do something simple like reading a book or going for a walk. We need to keep active in order to stay focused on our goals. Anything that allows you the opportunity to think about something else is what you need.

5 **Remember that there is more to life than food:** Yes, we need to eat and it is important to enjoy our food, but there are so many other things in your life. Sometimes when we allow our thoughts to take over we forget what is actually important. Try to hold on to what is really important in your life – whether it is family, friends or your job.

Achieving your five-a-day

You only have one body… take care of it. We are constantly being told about the importance of getting five portions of fruit and vegetables every day. The question is how many of us are actually doing it? Achieving your five-a-day might seem like a difficult goal if you are not inclined to eat fruit and vegetables on a regular basis. However, if you want to enjoy a healthy and balanced diet it is absolutely essential. Fruit and vegetables contain many of the nutrients we need and because they are low in calories you can eat plenty! They are also an excellent source of fibre and therefore good for healthy digestion. But how do we get into the habit of building fruit and vegetables into our daily routine? The answer lies in making sure that you include some portions with every meal and then you don't have to rely on getting your entire daily dose at dinnertime. The great thing about fruit and vegetables is that the options are endless, which means they are a great way of keeping your diet interesting. Just remember that potatoes are not included in your five-a-day as these are classed as a starchy food (see page 76).

- **Start the day well:** Get the day off to a fantastic start by having some fresh fruit with your breakfast. Porridge works well with blueberries, strawberries and bananas. Try out a few different varieties to decide which ones you prefer. Another way to enjoy fruit as part of your morning meal is to make some fresh juice – it's a great way of getting all the goodness out of fresh produce. If you don't feel like drinking it all first thing, take some of it with you to work. Alternatively, try some fresh fruit topped with Greek yogurt.

There are so many ways of incorporating fresh fruit and veg into your breakfast.

121

There are so many ways of incorporating fresh fruit and veg into your breakfast. If I am having poached or scrambled eggs for instance, I serve them with ripe tomatoes and mushrooms – not only do they add flavour, but I'm also having part of my five-a-day.

- **Have soup or salad for lunch:** Soup is one of the best ways to make sure you get a healthy portion of vegetables. Always try to make your own so that you can be sure it is packed with goodness (see page 148 for recipes). In winter, soup is a lovely comfort food as it warms us up! Choose from the huge variety of vegetables that are available to us, and flavour with garlic and pepper. If you make a large amount, soup can be frozen in the knowledge that it retains all of its original goodness.

  During the summer months, salads are the perfect alternative. Cucumber, tomatoes, beetroot, carrots and broccoli – the options are endless! Keep adding new items to your shopping list so that you never become bored (see pages 140–147 for recipes).

  If you are having an omelette for lunch, this is a good opportunity to include some vegetables. It's all about finding ways to include the five-a-day into your routine and the more you do it, the more it will become second nature.

- **Snack on fruit:** During the day you can eat a piece of fruit as a snack. Chop some apples or bring grapes in a container so that you can nibble on them during the day. Dried fruits are just as good for you as the fresh versions – raisins, apricots and figs are all good examples. Not only will they help you stay healthy, but also they should prevent you from reaching for the wrong types of snack during the day.

- **Have a stir-fry for dinner:** This is a brilliant way of ensuring that everyone is getting a vegetable-rich meal. Try baby corn, sugar snaps, bean sprouts, mange touts and red onions for variety. If you are serving a meal such as fish or chicken, make sure that you have your vegetable accompaniments or have a side salad.

Forget the tinned variety and make your own soup

Certain convenience foods are packaged in a way to make us believe that not only are they perfect for people on the go, but also that they contain some elements of goodness. Unfortunately, when it comes to tins or packets of soup, this isn't the case. It may seem like they are the easy option because all you have to do is pop them in the microwave or add some boiling water, but what you may not realise is just how bad they are for us. Often all we are taking in is more content with very little nutrition.

These types of soup contain large amounts of sodium. It's why many people find them so tasty, but often when you drink them you end up feeling incredibly thirsty. This level of salt is extremely unhealthy and should not be part of your daily diet. The other ingredient that many of these soups contain is MSG, otherwise known as monosodium glutamate, a food additive that enhances flavour. Although it is recognised as a safe ingredient, MSG has sparked controversy in the media and is widely thought of as something that should not form part of a healthy diet.

So how can you be sure that your soup contains no MSG or excess salt? Well, it all comes down to good old-fashioned home cooking! If you don't own a blender, now is the time to invest in one. One of the best things about homemade soup is that it retains the nutrients of the ingredients used. It fills you up and is full of goodness. Soup is easy to digest and the perfect low-fat option for your lunchtime meal. If you struggle to eat enough vegetables, making soup

> *If you don't own a blender, now is the time to invest in one.*

at home is a great way of including more in your diet.

When making your own soup, try to experiment with different ingredients. It's important to add a variety to your diet every day in order for your food to stay interesting, not something you are eating for the sake of it. There are so many recipes for vegetable soup, all of which are packed full of vitamins and minerals – from plain vegetable broth to carrot and ginger or spicy tomato. The great thing about homemade soup is that you can prepare a batch of it to use for the week ahead or freeze it to enjoy at a later date. All you need to know is that when it comes to soup, the only variety you should think of eating is one you have made yourself. Goodbye to that tinned variety; you can do so much better.

Swap time

One of the hardest challenges for many people will be cutting down on the sugary snacks that get them through the day. Whether it's the biscuits with your coffee at eleven, the crisps you grab at lunchtime or the mid-afternoon chocolate treat that gets you through the slump at work, you are not on your own! Many people find these habits extremely hard to break. We get used to having certain snacks at certain times of the day and fear our body will go into shock if it doesn't get them. Well, let me tell you straight out that you will survive. This is coming from the woman who once enjoyed a half packet of biscuits with my morning cappuccino! If I can do it, so can you. There are plenty of healthier and tastier snacks out there – trust me, they are tasty! Say goodbye to your chocolate digestives and salty crisps: it's swap time!

- **Swap your digestive for a homemade granola bar:** Even if we start the day with a good breakfast, many of us still find ourselves reaching for the biscuit tin by eleven o'clock. If you are usually a biscuit fan, now is the time to get out of that routine and find an alternative – because, let's be honest, the majority of us find it hard to stop at one biscuit! Reality check for you: a plain digestive biscuit contains on average 75kcal and 3g fat. So, by munching more than one you can see how much damage you are doing. Instead, you need to swap your digestive for one of the breakfast biscuits on the market, which on average contain half the calories and half the fat. Alternatively, have a rice cake. Or go a step further and make your own flapjacks or granola bars (see page 138 for a recipe). If you make them yourself, you can control exactly what goes into the mixture. Just make sure you bring them to work with you to avoid temptation in the canteen.

• **Swap crisps for walnuts, almonds or chestnuts:** If you regularly reach for a packet of crisps, let's kick this habit to the curb. Crisps are so bad for you and they are incredibly addictive. It's hard to have only one or two. On average, a packet of cheese and onion crisps contains 170kcal and an incredible 11g fat. While I don't think it's healthy to become obsessed by food labels, I do believe that sometimes it does no harm to be confronted by the facts. Now that you know what crisps contain, it's easy to see why your daily diet is better without them. The alternative to this salty snack is nuts. Nuts are rich in protein and fill you up quite quickly. Opt for walnuts, almonds or chestnuts, as these are low in fat as well. Limit your portion to no more than a handful and try to spread it out over the day, so that if you feel peckish you always have something to reach for.

• **Stock up on carrot and celery sticks:** One of the times we often find ourselves craving sugary or salty snacks is when we have a glass of wine. My tip here would be to forget the nachos, as these are a recipe for a diet disaster! Instead stock up on carrot and celery sticks that work really well with low-fat hummus dip. Hummus is a great healthy snack because it's made with chickpeas, which are low in fat and a good source of fibre. By eating carrots and celery you are also getting two of your five-a-day, so it's a no-brainer!

There is more to life than food!

- **Beat that afternoon slump with dried apricots or blueberries:** When you hit three o'clock in the afternoon and feel desperate for a bar of chocolate, just stop yourself. If it means avoiding the canteen or the vending machine where temptation lies, that's what you need to do. Think about it logically: you will be eating an evening meal in a couple of hours, so you don't need a sugary snack at this time. Try having some dried apricots or blueberries instead, which will satisfy the need for something sweet without piling on the pounds.

Every aspect of your diet needs to change and fooling yourself into thinking you are eating healthily is the biggest mistake that people make. Everything you do comes down to a choice that you make. I'm trying to encourage you to make the right one; however, I can't do it for you. Eating well at mealtimes and then snacking on the wrong foods in between will never work. Eating well is part of your lifestyle now. Each time you do your weekly shop you need to keep this mentality. You can lose weight and still enjoy what you eat. It just means making changes and being open to trying new things.

When you're eating well, occasionally 'falling off the wagon' does no harm

As you find your way with your new lifestyle there will be times when you feel like throwing caution to the wind and eating everything in sight! It's still normal to crave treats and if you can manage to keep things on track for the majority of the time, the odd outburst will do you no harm. I think the worst thing you can do is become obsessed with every single detail of what you eat. Doing this often leads to overeating as you spend so much time thinking about food. Depriving yourself is not the answer. The reason why many people fail on diets is that they try to go without too much and end up giving in to temptation before eventually giving up. Improving your health is what's important and this is about eating well most of the time. You are entitled to a day off, so make sure you take it.

The one thing I noticed when I changed my ways was that I really enjoyed the switch to healthy food, and I genuinely started to feel better in myself. You have to do it to believe me! Gone were my biscuits in the morning and the chocolate bar in the afternoon. As time went by the old eating habits that I loved were replaced by good alternatives. I can honestly say that today I no longer want to eat what I did before. My body has become used to eating foods that are actually better for me. However, this took time and your body won't adjust immediately, which is why I feel strongly about the importance of letting go occasionally and not depriving yourself all the time.

How to treat yourself without losing control
Here are some things you can do to rein in your eating on a day off:

 If you decide to have a day off, the best advice I can give is to enjoy it – otherwise, what is the point of treating yourself? Don't feel guilty. Live in the moment. Put it behind you the next day and move on.

 Try not to eat to the point where you feel unwell. This means you have overeaten. Enjoy the food without making yourself uncomfortable. Take your time and eat slowly.

 Don't talk about it too much, just do it! Sometimes when people are trying to lose weight they spend more time talking about it than acting on it. If you're having a day off from your diet, that's nobody's business but yours.

 Treat yourself to the foods you really want. Don't eat for the sake of it. Always remember to listen to your body.

 Don't let it throw you off the healthy eating plan. Enjoy it at the time, but make sure that your overall eating habits are still the best that they can be.

You don't need to deny yourself all the time!

Chapter nine

Recipes for HEALTHY, DELICIOUS FOOD

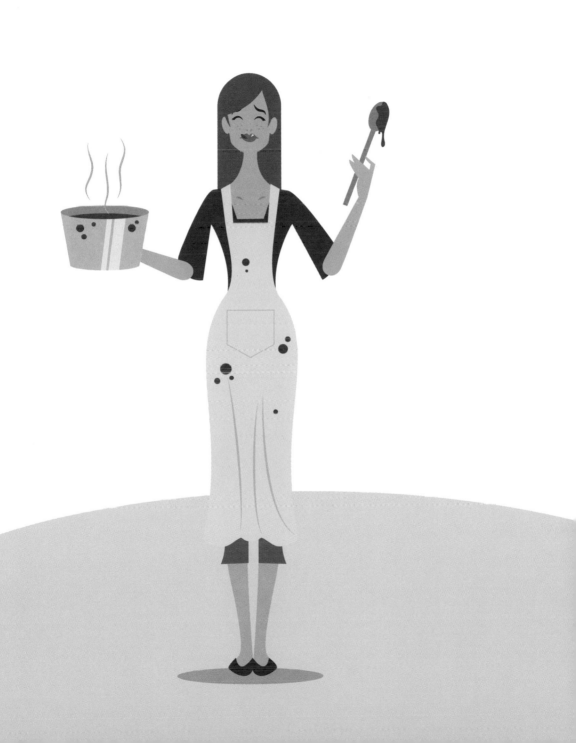

Breakfast

Poached eggs with cherry tomatoes

| 11.4g **fat** | 3.0g **saturates** | 1.7g **sugars** | 0.38g **salt** | **162 calories** |

Poached eggs are a firm favourite in our house! High in protein and Vitamin D, they are such a great way to start the day. Cherry tomatoes are the perfect accompaniment – naturally high in fibre and a good source of Vitamin C.

1 tablespoon white wine vinegar
2 free-range eggs
6 cherry tomatoes
sprig of parsley, chopped
freshly ground black pepper

1. Half-fill a pan with water, add the vinegar and bring to the boil. Once the water comes to the boil, reduce the heat to low.
2. Break the eggs into a small cup. Swirl the water in the pan to create a whirlpool effect and gently slide the eggs into the centre, making sure they are well separated. Cook for approx. 3 minutes.
3. Meanwhile cut the cherry tomatoes in half and grill under a moderate heat for 2–3 minutes.
4. To serve, remove the poached eggs from the pan with a slotted spoon and transfer them to a serving plate with the grilled tomatoes. Garnish with parsley and season with black pepper.

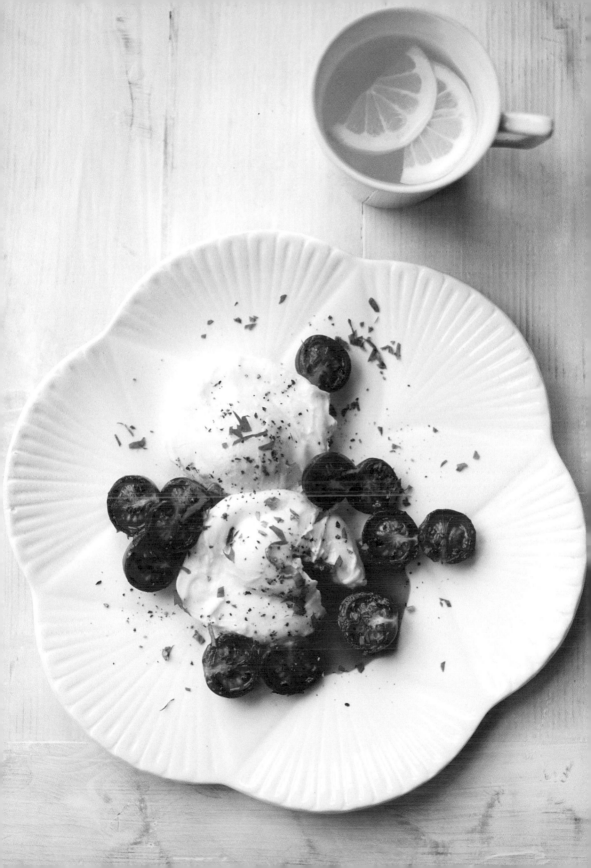

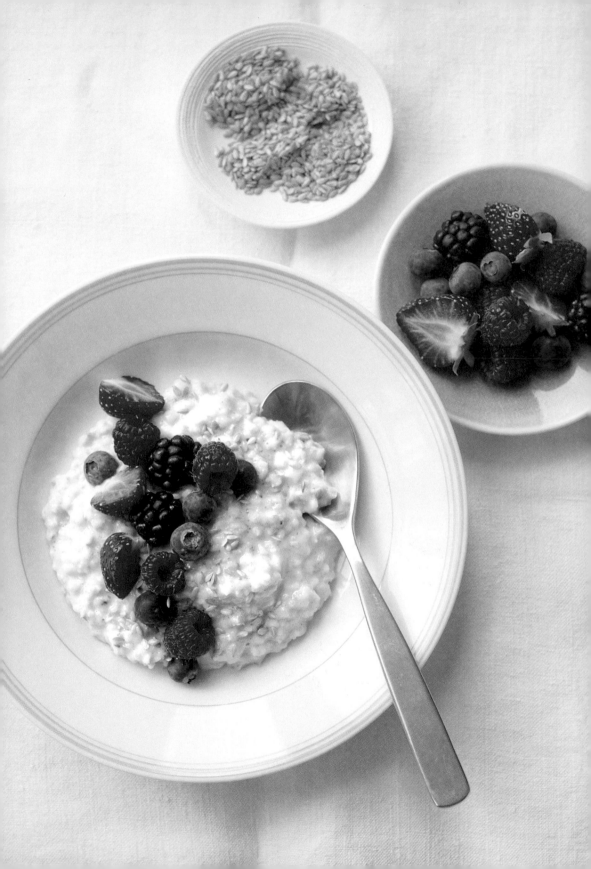

Porridge with soya milk and fresh berries

| 11.9g **fat** | 1.6g **saturates** | 5.8g **sugars** | 0.21g **salt** | **314 calories** |

Eating porridge first thing in the morning gives you slow releasing energy, because oats take longer to digest than many breakfast cereals. Prepared with soya milk (which is much lower in saturated fat than regular milk) and berries you are staying healthy but not loosing out on taste!

50g organic oat flakes
225ml soya milk
2 handfuls of fresh berries
1 tablespoon flax seeds

1. Place the oat flakes and soya milk in a saucepan and bring to the boil. Reduce the heat to low and cook for 5–6 minutes, stirring constantly to prevent sticking.
2. Pour into a bowl and serve with some fresh berries and a sprinkling of flax seeds.

Soya yogurt with fresh berries and granola

| 14.2g **fat** | 1.3g **saturates** | 34.9g **sugars** | 0.13g **salt** | **497 calories** |

Eating granola is a brilliant way of filling up on whole grains and is a great source of fibre. Along with the nutritious soya yogurt it's an ideal alternative to the traditional breakfast cereal and is bursting with flavour.

100g granola
125g pot soya yogurt
75g fresh berries

1. Place half the granola in a parfait glass and top with half the yogurt. Repeat the layers and top with the fresh berries.

Berry smoothie

| 1.4g **fat** | 0.7g **saturates** | 27.8g **sugars** | 0.07g **salt** | **140 calories** |

When you are on the go this is the perfect option. It's easy to make and the antioxidants in berries are so good for you. The natural yogurt gives it a lovely flavour and is a good way to increase your calcium intake.

4 tablespoons blueberries
4 tablespoons raspberries
1 banana, peeled
2 tablespoons natural yogurt

1. Place the fruit in a blender and blitz to a smooth purée.
2. Stir in the yogurt and serve immediately.

Egg-white omelette with avocado

| 41.1g **fat** | 8.4g **saturates** | 1.0g **sugars** | 0.34g **salt** | **423 calories** |

I love this because you are getting all the benefits of an egg but with lower cholesterol content. The avocado is rich in monounsaturated fat, which is important for our cholesterol.

1 teaspoon olive oil   **freshly ground black pepper**
2 free-range egg whites   **1 large avocado, peeled, stoned and sliced**
1 teaspoon soya milk

1. Heat a non-stick frying pan over a medium heat and add the olive oil.
2. Combine the egg whites and soya milk in a bowl and whisk together lightly. Season with a little black pepper.
3. Pour the egg mixture into the hot pan, tilting it backwards and forwards so that the egg spreads out evenly. Using a fork, drag the cooked egg from the outside towards the middle of the pan so that the uncooked egg spreads around evenly to fill any gaps.
4. Once the egg is almost set, scatter over the slices of avocado, fold the omelette in half to enclose the filling and quickly slide onto a plate. Season with a little more black pepper to taste.

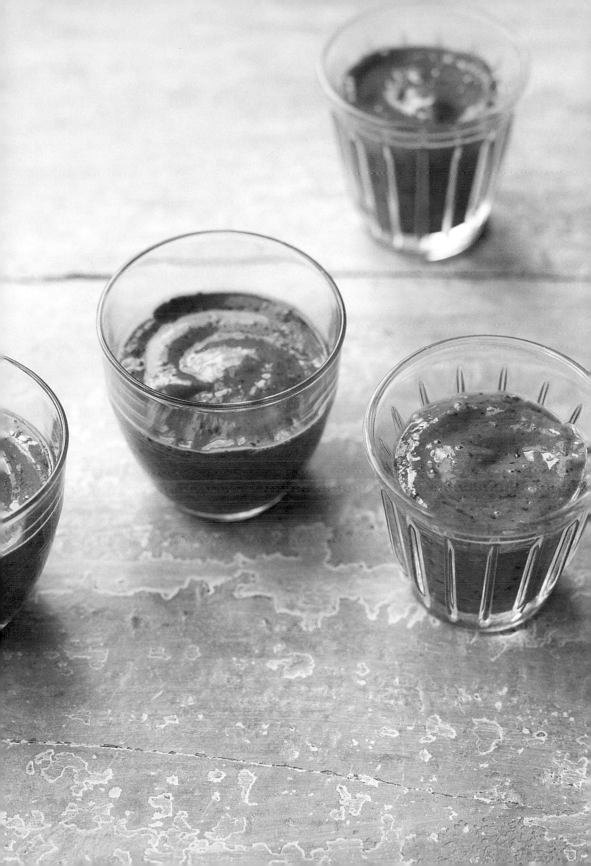

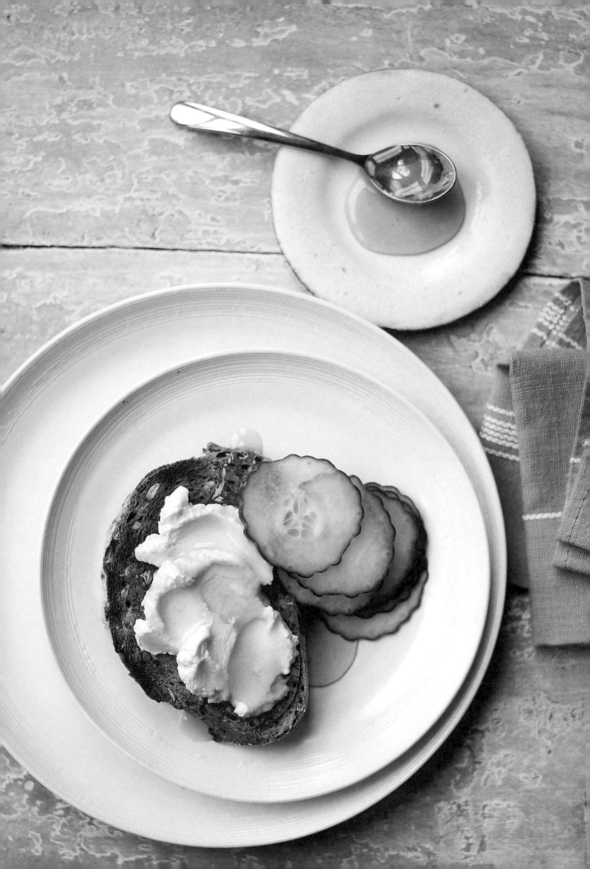

Wholegrain toast with ricotta and honey

| 6.5g fat | 3.6g **saturates** | 13.7g **sugars** | 0.36g **salt** | **203 calories** |

When it comes to choosing a cheese that is low in fat and doesn't compromise on taste, ricotta is a great option. It works so well with the honey, toast and cucumber on the side.

1 slice of wholegrain bread
2 heaped tablespoons ricotta
1 tablespoon honey
6 thin slices of cucumber

1. Toast the bread and spread with the ricotta.
2. Drizzle over the honey and garnish with the cucumber slices.

Healthy granola bar

| 7.0g **fat** | 1.0g **saturates** | 6.3g **sugars** | 0.02g **salt** | **145 calories** |

I have learned to perfect these over the years, as the kids love them! They are a super morning snack or, if you don't have time to sit down for breakfast, pop one in your bag. They also contain manuka honey, which is known to aid digestion, boost the immune system and provide you with energy.

200g organic oat flakes
115ml unsweetened apple juice
75g whole almonds
55g pumpkin seeds
75g dried apricots/raisins
2 tablespoons manuka honey

1. Preheat the oven to 150°C/gas mark 2 and line a 20 x 30cm baking tray with greaseproof paper. Place all the ingredients in a mixing bowl and mix well with a wooden spoon until well combined.
2. Spoon the mixture into the prepared baking tray and spread out in an even layer. Bake in the oven for approx. 10 minutes until the top has turned golden brown.

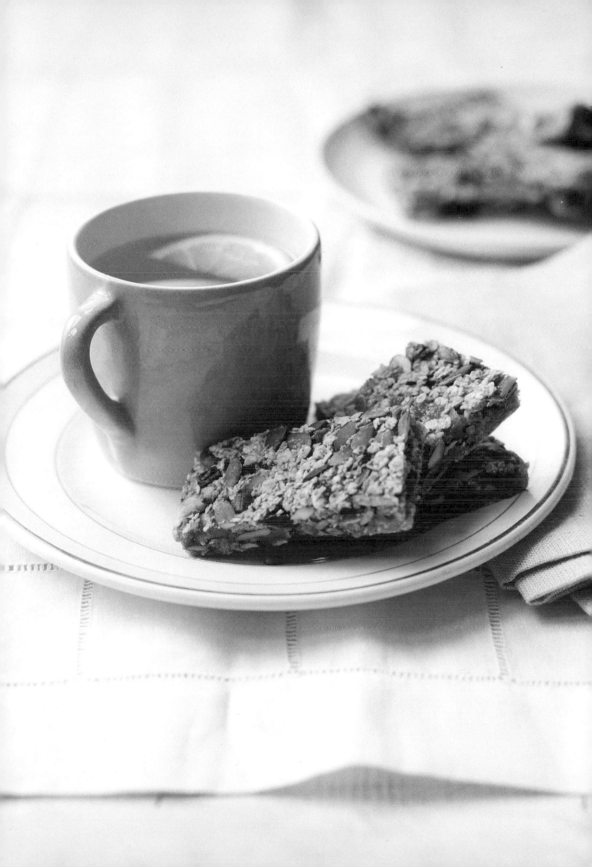

Lunch

Beetroot and goat's cheese salad

| 10.9g **fat** | 3.4g **saturates** | 13.8g **sugars** | 0.63g **salt** | **189 calories** |

The combination of beetroot and goat's cheese is one that has to be tried to be believed! Beetroot is a fantastic source of iron, vitamins and contains antioxidant properties, so this recipe ticks all the right boxes.

1 large cooked beetroot, cut into 3 slices
15g goat's cheese, cut into 3 slices
a handful of rocket
1 tablespoon balsamic vinegar
1 tablespoon pine nuts

1. Top the 3 slices of beetroot with the 3 slices of goat's cheese and place under a moderate grill until the cheese is bubbling and golden brown.
2. Arrange on a bed of fresh rocket, drizzle with the balsamic vinegar and garnish with the pine nuts.

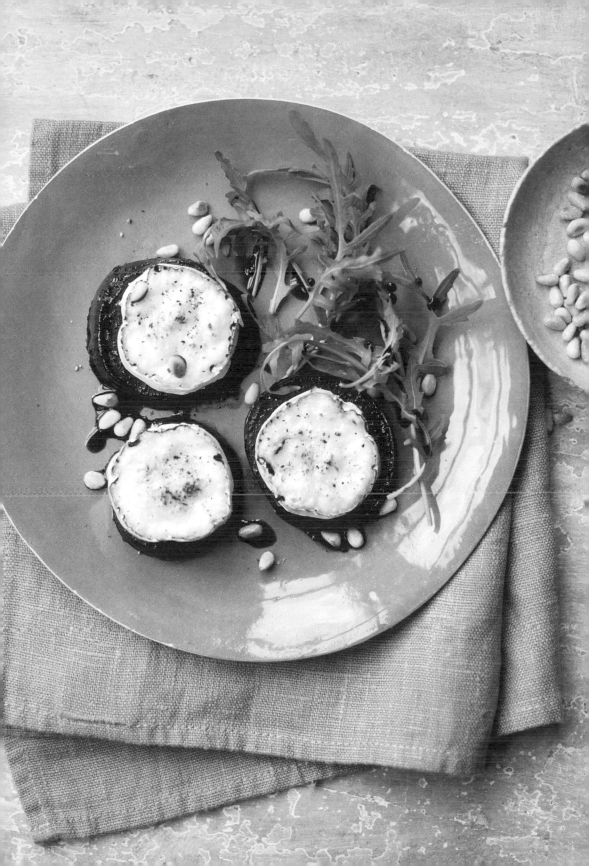

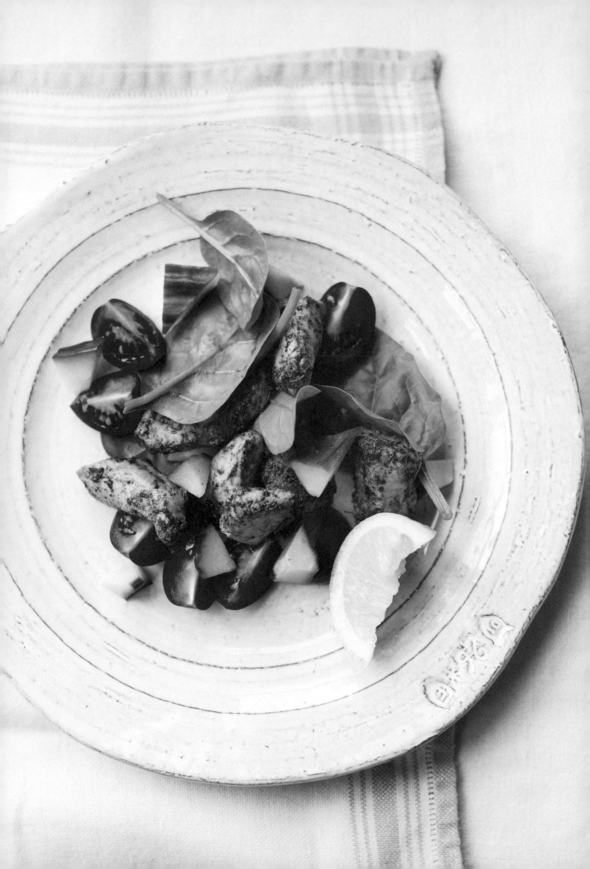

Cajun chicken salad

13.0g **fat**   1.4g **saturates**   1.8g **sugars**   0.74g **salt**   **270 calories**

This is one of the easiest and tastiest salads you can make. The Cajun spice is full of flavour and the spinach is packed with nutrients, which make it the perfect choice for a light lunch.

1 organic chicken breast
2 teaspoons olive oil
2 tablespoons Cajun seasoning
a large handful of baby spinach leaves
4 cherry tomatoes, quartered
a handful of chopped cucumber
1 lemon wedge, to serve

1. Preheat the oven to 180°C/gas mark 4. Cut the chicken breast into bite-sized pieces and mix with the olive oil and Cajun seasoning in a bowl.
2. Transfer to an ovenproof dish and bake in the oven for 20 minutes or until cooked through.
3. Prepare the salad by mixing together the baby spinach leaves, cherry tomatoes and cucumber.
4. Remove the chicken from the oven and toss it through the salad. Serve straight away, accompanied by the lemon wedge, for squeezing.

Mixed bean salad

| 29.8g **fat** | 4.0g **saturates** | 9.7g **sugars** | 0.28g **salt** | **598 calories** |

One of the best things about mixed beans is that they are so versatile. They are rich in protein and high in fibre. The vegetables included in this recipe mean you are also helping with that all-important five-a-day!

100g dried mixed beans
4 sugar snap peas
4 French beans
3 radishes
4 cherry tomatoes
¼ red onion
a handful of sunflower seeds

For the dressing
2 tablespoons olive oil
1 tablespoon balsamic vinegar
½ teaspoon mustard

1. Soak the beans in cold water overnight; drain.
2. Cover the beans with fresh cold water and simmer over a moderate heat for 20 minutes. Drain and allow to cool.
3. Meanwhile, chop the sugar snap peas, French beans and radishes. Halve the cherry tomatoes and finely chop the red onion.
4. To make the salad dressing, place the olive oil, vinegar and mustard in an empty jar. Put on the lid and shake well.
5. To serve, combine all the salad ingredients in a bowl, pour over the dressing and sprinkle with the sunflower seeds.

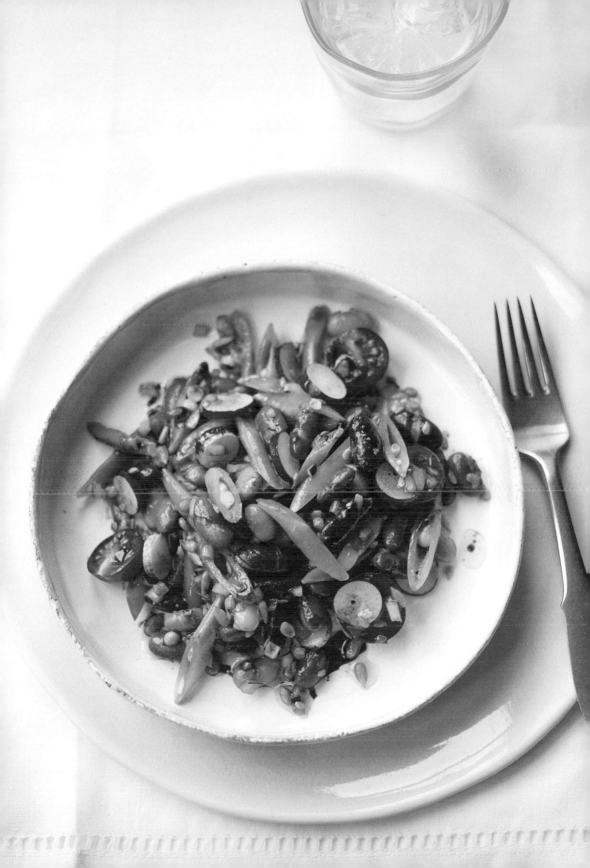

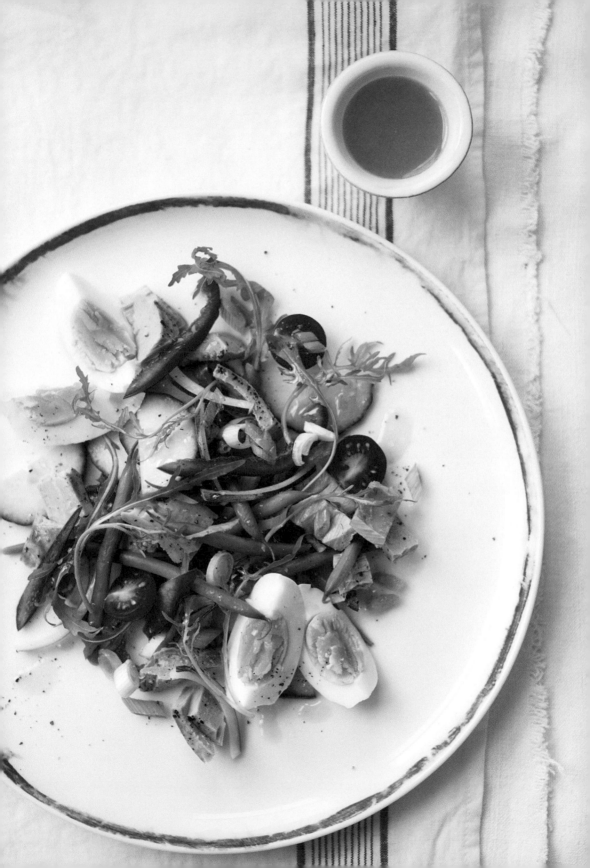

Healthy salad Niçoise

| 30.3g **fat** | 5.5g **saturates** | 20.9g **sugars** | 0.59g **salt** | **557 calories** |

I have always been a fan of salad niçoise. Whilst this is a healthy version it certainly doesn't let us down when it comes to flavour. Tuna steak is one of the best sources of omega-3 and it also contains lots of essential nutrients.

150g fresh tuna steak
freshly ground black pepper
1 egg, hard-boiled and shelled
1 spring onion, chopped
1 red onion, finely chopped
1 red pepper, deseeded and sliced
6 slices of cucumber, chopped
4 cherry tomatoes
a handful of green beans
a handful of rocket

For the dressing
1½ tablespoon olive oil
1 tablespoon balsamic vinegar
½ teaspoon mustard

1. Season the tuna steak with black pepper and place under a moderate grill for approx. 6 minutes, turning once during grilling. Set aside to cool.
2. Prepare all of the salad ingredients and arrange them in a bowl.
3. To make the salad dressing, place the olive oil, vinegar and mustard in an empty jar. Put on the lid and shake well.
4. Cut the tuna into strips and arrange on the salad. Drizzle over the salad dressing to serve.

Carrot and lentil soup

| 14.9g **fat** | 1.7g **saturates** | 32.4g **sugars** | 2.59g **salt** | **565 calories** |

This is a real winter warmer, packed full of goodness. Low in fat and with plenty of iron and protein. My advice is to make this your go-to comfort soup!

1 tablespoon olive oil	85g red lentils
1 small onion, finely chopped	2 large carrots, chopped
2 garlic cloves, crushed	½ x 425g tin of chopped tomatoes
1 teaspoon chilli flakes	200ml vegetable stock
1 teaspoon garam masala	salt and freshly ground black pepper to taste

1. Heat the oil in a medium saucepan over a high heat. Add the onion and garlic and cook for 5 minutes until soft.
2. Add the chilli flakes and garam masala and cook for 1 minute, stirring.
3. Put in the rest of the ingredients and bring to the boil, stirring. Turn down the heat and simmer until the lentils are soft, approx. 20 minutes.
4. Remove from the heat and use a hand-held blender to purée the soup. Season to taste with salt and black pepper.

Tomato, beetroot and celery soup

| 0.9g **fat** | 0.1g **saturates** | 22.7g **sugars** | 0.79g **salt** | **146 calories** |

If you are looking to fill up on the very best of vegetables with vitamins and minerals then this is the one for you. I love making a big pot and keeping it in the fridge for a few days. This soup can be served hot or cold.

425g tin of chopped tomatoes	1 medium onion, finely chopped
250ml cold water	1 teaspoon lemon juice
1 small uncooked beetroot, scrubbed and roughly chopped	2 bay leaves
1 celery stick, roughly chopped	freshly ground black pepper

1. Place all the ingredients in a large saucepan and simmer over a medium heat until the vegetables are cooked, approx. 25 minutes.
2. Remove the bay leaves and blitz to a purée using a hand-held blender.

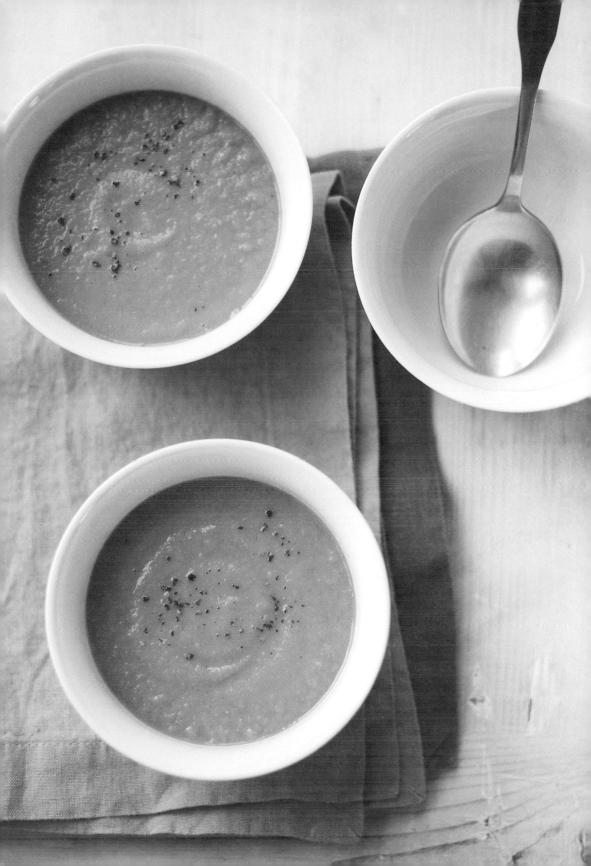

Dinner

Lemon basil sea bass with brown rice

| 17.7g **fat** | 2.9g **saturates** | 2.2g **sugars** | 0.40g **salt** | **591 calories** |

Sea bass is a real treat for dinner at home. It's rich in protein and omega-3. Brown rice is chewier and has a nuttier flavour than the white variety. It's also better for us because all of the natural nutrients are kept.

100g brown basmati rice
150g sea bass fillet
freshly ground black pepper
½ lemon
a handful of basil leaves
1 tablespoon olive oil

1. Preheat the oven to 180°C/gas mark 4. Place the rice in a saucepan with 250ml water. Bring to the boil, reduce the heat and simmer until all the liquid has been absorbed and the rice is cooked, approx. 25–30 minutes.
2. Season the fish with black pepper and transfer to an ovenproof dish. Cut off 3 thin slices of lemon and place them on top of the fish along with the basil. Squeeze the rest of the lemon juice over the fish and drizzle with the olive oil.
3. Transfer the fish to the oven and bake for 8 minutes until the fish is cooked through.
4. Carefully lift the fish onto a plate, pour the cooking juices over the top and serve with the brown rice.

Chicken stir-fry

38.1g **fat**   4.8g **saturates**   19.6g **sugars**   3.05g **salt**   **642 calories**

I've tried so many variations of chicken stir-fry and always come back to this one. It's the mix of vegetables with the organic chicken that makes it work so well. The cashew nuts also give it extra flavour and have plenty of protein.

1 tablespoon olive oil
1 organic chicken breast, cut into bite-sized pieces
2 garlic cloves, finely chopped
2 tablespoons finely chopped fresh root ginger
1 red pepper, deseeded and sliced
1 green pepper, deseeded and sliced
a handful of sugar snap peas
a handful of baby corn
50g cashew nuts
1 tablespoon light soy sauce

1. Heat the oil in a wok and stir-fry the chicken breast for 5 minutes until cooked through.
2. Add the garlic and ginger and cook for a further 2 minutes.
3. Add the peppers, sugar snap peas, baby corn, cashew nuts and soy sauce. Stir-fry until the vegetables are tender, being careful not to overcook.
4. Serve immediately.

Vegetarian lasagne

11.2g **fat**	3.7g **saturates**	18.3g **sugars**	0.65g **salt**	**496 calories**

The great news is that just because you are following a healthy plan doesn't mean you can't have pasta! This is a twist on the traditional lasagne but is every bit as tasty. Lentils are low in fat, great for our digestive system and are a good source of protein. Use wholewheat pasta as it is unprocessed and is the most nutritious variety.

Serves 4

250g dried green lentils

2 teaspoons olive oil

1 large onion, chopped

2 garlic cloves, crushed to a paste

1 aubergine, diced

1 courgette, sliced

1 red pepper, deseeded and chopped

425g tin of chopped tomatoes

1 tablespoon tomato purée

freshly ground black pepper

8 sheets of non pre-cook wholewheat lasagne

50g low-fat Cheddar cheese, grated

For the white sauce

300ml natural yogurt

2 free-range eggs

1. Preheat the oven to 180°C/gas mark 4. Place the green lentils in a saucepan and cover with cold water. Bring to the boil and cook, uncovered, for 10 minutes. Now reduce the heat, cover with a lid and simmer for a further 20 minutes.
2. Meanwhile, heat the oil in a large saucepan and fry the onion and garlic for 5 minutes until soft.
3. Add the aubergine, courgette and red pepper and cook for a further 10 minutes.
4. Tip in the tomatoes, add the tomato purée and season with black pepper. Continue to cook for a further 5 minutes, stirring occasionally, until the mixture is cooked through.
5. Drain the cooked lentils and combine them with the vegetables.
6. To assemble the dish, cover the base of an ovenproof dish with a thin layer of the vegetable filling. Cover with a layer of lasagne sheets and repeat the layers until the filling and lasagne have been used up, finishing with a layer of lasagne.
7. To make the white sauce, combine the yogurt with the eggs in a mixing bowl and beat well together. Pour the sauce over the lasagne and sprinkle with the grated cheese.
8. Bake in the oven for approx. 40 minutes until the topping is golden brown.

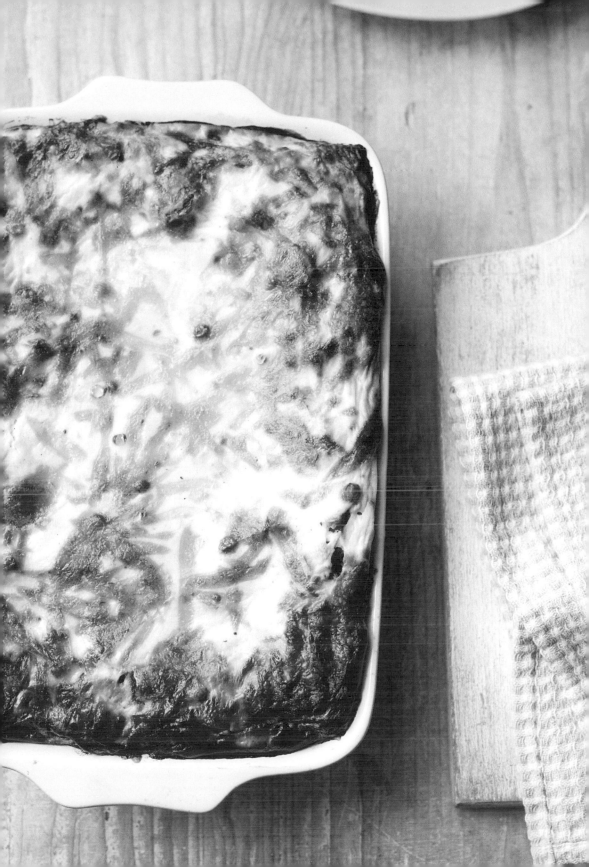

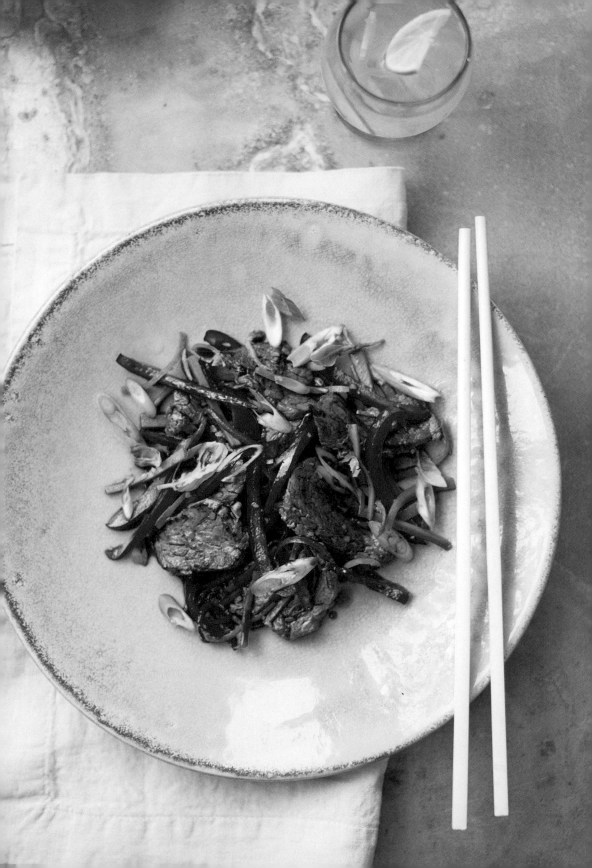

Thai beef stir-fry

| 16.5g **fat** | 3.3g **saturates** | 24.5g **sugars** | 3.44g **salt** | **364 calories** |

Trust me, this is as good as you would get in any restaurant. Increase your iron intake with some tasty lean beef and enjoy the gorgeous flavours of ginger and spring onions mixed with chilli and other vegetables.

1 tablespoon olive oil

100g lean beef steak, cut into thin strips

1 garlic clove, crushed

2.5cm piece of fresh root ginger, peeled and sliced

1 red chilli, deseeded and chopped

1 red pepper, deseeded and thinly sliced

1 carrot, thinly sliced

4 spring onions, chopped

2 tablespoons oyster sauce

a handful of basil leaves, shredded

1. Heat a wok over a high heat and pour in the oil. Add the beef and stir-fry over a high heat for 2–3 minutes. Remove the meat from the pan and transfer it to a plate to keep warm.
2. Return the pan to a low heat and add the garlic, ginger and chilli. Stir-fry for approx. 1 minute to release their flavours, then pour in 2–3 tablespoons water.
3. Increase the heat, add the red pepper, carrot and spring onions and fry together for approx. 2 minutes.
4. Return the beef to the wok, pour in the oyster sauce and simmer for a further 1 minute. Garnish with the basil and serve immediately.

Oven-baked salmon with brown basmati rice

| 22.6g **fat** | 4.2g **saturates** | 3.1g **sugars** | 0.29g **salt** | **584 calories** |

Oven-baked salmon is delicious and simple to make if you are having people over. The salmon is so tasty when cooked this way and is a source of both protein and Vitamin D. Broccoli contains a large amount of calcium, B vitamins and iron.

150g salmon fillet
1 teaspoon olive oil
3 slices of lemon
75g brown basmati rice
a handful of broccoli florets
a sprig of flat-leaf parsley, chopped, to garnish

1. Preheat the oven to 180°C/gas mark 4. Place the salmon in a roasting dish, drizzle with the oil and arrange the lemon slices on top. Cover with aluminium foil and bake in the oven for 15 minutes.
2. Meanwhile, cook the basmati rice according to the instructions on the packet.
3. Steam the broccoli until tender.
4. To serve, arrange the salmon on a plate, garnish with the flat-leaf parsley and accompany with the rice and broccoli.

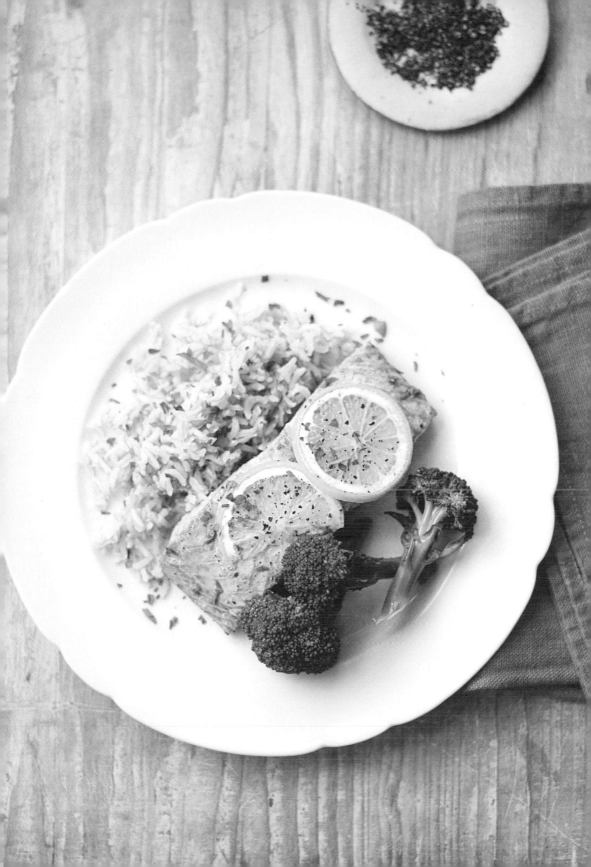

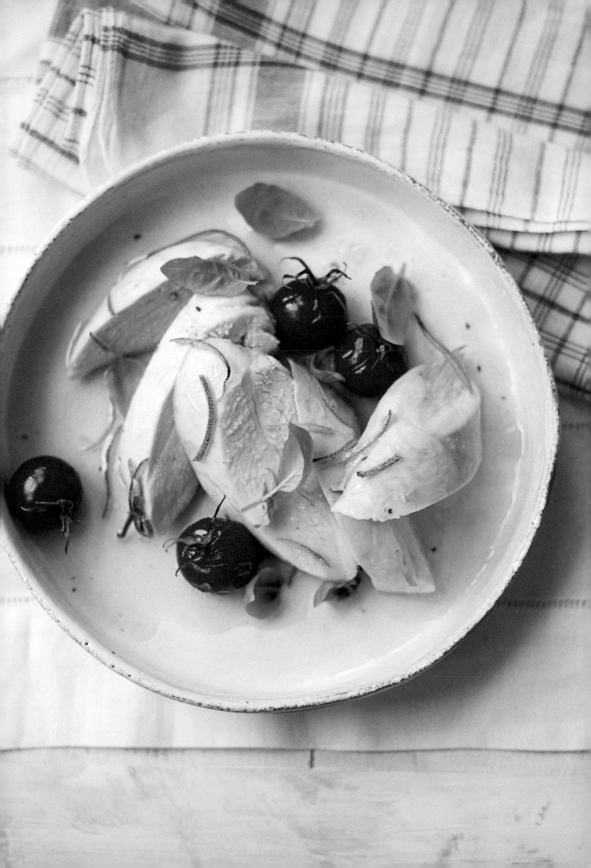

Lime chicken with cherry tomatoes and basil

12.6g **fat**   2.0g **saturates**   14.6g **sugars**   0.21g **salt**   **294 calories**

If you're looking for something a little different when it comes to cooking chicken, you have to try this. The cherry tomatoes are high in Vitamin C and a good source of Vitamin E. Served with the lime chicken and basil, this is a fresh-tasting dish.

juice and grated zest of 1 lime
1 tablespoon manuka honey
1 tablespoon olive oil
1 organic chicken breast
4 cherry tomatoes
a handful of basil leaves

1. Preheat the oven to 180°C/gas mark 4. To make a marinade, mix together the lime juice and zest, honey and oil in a bowl. Pour the mixture over the chicken and transfer to a roasting tin.
2. Roast the chicken in the oven for approx. 25 minutes, and then throw in the tomatoes and cook for a further 5 minutes
3. To serve, slice the chicken and transfer to a plate with the tomatoes, then scatter over the basil leaves.

Chapter ten

Maintaining
YOUR WEIGHT LOSS

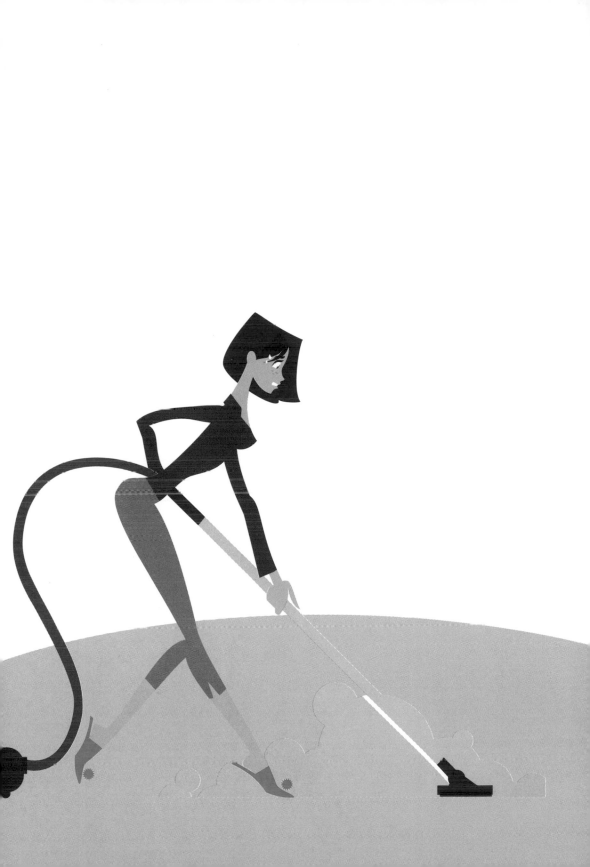

> *Don't leave the house in the morning without the food that you have prepared.*

So you're sailing along and making huge progress on the road to a new and improved lifestyle. You're eating better, feeling healthier and moving around so much more. You think to yourself, 'I'm getting the hang of this now!' I remember that feeling very well.

It's an incredible time when you actually start to lose weight. Suddenly you feel better in yourself and you believe that you are achieving something that seemed impossible before. You start to notice a difference when you look in the mirror. Even though it's a small change, it's still important. However, this is a point in your journey you need to be prepared for. I can recall the day when I tried on something in my wardrobe and realised that a wonderful thing had happened. It was too big for me! I was excited, happy and proud all at the same time. My hard work was starting to pay off and I could see the results for myself. So what happened next? Did I continue my journey as before? No, I had a little slip-up because I thought that if my clothes were too big, I had earned the right to eat what I wanted. Big mistake…

If you want to turn your life around for good, you have to stick to the plan, ladies! Don't leave the house in the morning without the food that you have prepared. Always be aware of what you're eating and try to make healthy choices. Enjoy your food and really taste it. Be conscious of your portion sizes and try not to overeat. Carry your bottle of water with you. You know all this already, so it's just a gentle reminder! Get back on track and keep going. You're doing just fine. Keep your eye on the prize, which is to lose weight and feel healthy.

Surviving Christmas while losing weight

Christmas is an amazing time of the year. Well, I think it is anyway – I absolutely love getting into the festive spirit and seeing the kids enjoying themselves. But for many of us ladies it can also bring with it a certain amount of stress. In general, the women seem to be in charge of making sure that everything is just right. Present buying, decorating the house, cooking the dinner, our list goes on for quite a while. Then you throw into the mix the fact that you are now on the road to losing weight. You're panicking and wondering how you can survive it, keep your sanity and not pile on the pounds. But at the same time you want to enjoy Christmas and not be paranoid about every single piece of food that passes your lips. The first thing to do is not let it get you down. You are entitled to enjoy Christmas like everybody else. It stands to reason that if you have taken all the steps so far to lose weight, you don't want to undo all your hard work. There will probably be nights out and in over the Christmas period that involve mince pies, canapés, nibbles and alcohol. Rest assured, you don't have to run scared every time you see a platter of food coming your way! Take a deep breath, don't worry and follow some simple guidelines, which will help you to stay in control and still enjoy the holiday.

- **Breakfast:** Make sure that you start the day as you always do with a healthy breakfast. Starving yourself in order to save calories to gorge on later will just have the wrong effect. Chances are you will be much more likely to overindulge when you do eat. If you can have some protein with your breakfast this will help to keep you full for longer. Scrambled eggs and smoked salmon are a perfect mix to keep you going.

- **Parties:** If you find yourself at the office party or at a family night out where there is food everywhere, there are simple things that you can do to help. Eating slowly is a great tip – you don't have to dive into everything that's on your plate! Take your time and give yourself a chance to digest the food – you are more likely to enjoy it as well. Allow yourself time to register when you're full. As I've said before, we often don't give our body a chance to tell us when we have had enough: we just keep eating. Take a break in between bites and see how you feel. You'll probably surprise yourself and realise that you're full more quickly than you thought you'd be. It is actually OK to leave food on the plate; you don't have to finish every single thing in front of you. Enjoying your food at Christmas doesn't mean stuffing your face and feeling uncomfortable. If you are worried about how much you are eating, and think it might be getting out of control, keep a food diary (see page 110). This will help you to watch what you're consuming; it's a great reality check and should help to get you back on track.

- **Alcohol:** As you know, when it comes to alcohol you are dealing with empty calories, so do your best to keep an eye on the amount that you're drinking – not an easy task at Christmas when we are constantly confronted with temptation. Try to eat before you have a drink, to give your food a chance to digest. Be aware of mixers and stick to soda or tonic water. The good news for fans of mulled wine is that it's rich in antioxidants and because it has been heated the alcohol content is reduced. If you're worried about your intake around this time, try the water trick: for every drink of alcohol, sip a glass of water. You'll find yourself drinking less and your head will be clearer in the morning!

- **Christmas dinner:** On Christmas day, you will probably find that you eat more than you do on other days. Well, this is an understatement if statistics are anything to go by. Research has shown that the average person consumes a staggering 4,000–7,000 calories on 25 December! Fry-ups, huge dinners, sandwiches, nibbles, sweets and wine mean that you are less likely to press the 'stop' button on this special day! However, now that you are on the road to weight loss you can still indulge a little without doing damage. Just don't lose sight of all that you have achieved and try to make healthy choices – for example, fill up on turkey rather than roast potatoes. It's a great source of protein and it will fill you up. Brussels sprouts can be quite controversial, but they are packed with fibre and vitamin C, so if you can manage to eat them it's worthwhile!

Now you're on the road to weight loss you can still indulge without doing damage.

Enjoying the summer holidays

Your bags are all packed and you are ready to go on your summer holidays with your family or you have simply taken a week off to rest. It's the time of year when rules seem to fly out the window. The kids go to bed a little later and your wine glass is a little fuller than usual! Food is everywhere and, to make matters worse, everything comes in huge portions. How could you possibly resist? It would be rude to say no. We all know the pattern: when that tiny bit of guilt starts to creep in we casually brush it off, reminding ourselves that we are on holiday, we deserve it. Of course, you have worked hard and you do need to let your hair down once in a while – that's only normal – but it doesn't mean you have to throw the rule book out of the window and make no attempt to retrieve it. I try my best to be as true to my healthy lifestyle as I can while I'm on holiday, but of course I also have some fun along the way. Here are my top tips for surviving that all-important summer break, staying sane and still having a glass or two of vino!

 Eat a good breakfast: It's easy to be tempted by a greasy fry-up or buttery croissants and pastries, but eating those every day will inevitably have consequences. Try to start your day with some poached eggs or fresh fruit and yogurt. If you eat well first thing in the morning, you are less likely to pick at food throughout the day.

 Don't forget the exercise: Wherever you are, my advice would be to keep that body working. If you have access to a gym, swimming pool or even the sea, make use of it first thing in the morning. Alternatively, take yourself out for a walk. It doesn't really matter what you do – just don't let your muscles go into hibernation!

 Remember to check in on your body: You can still ask yourself the question, 'Am I hungry?' This will stop you from eating mindlessly and just for the sake of it. It's easy to forget this when you are out of your routine, so best to be aware of it.

 Keep an eye on portions: It's OK to be a bit more relaxed about the food you're eating, but be careful of the amount. Do your best to practise portion control and, if you can, eat from a smaller plate. It's a great trick and it works well.

You can't eat foods you enjoy and it seems like the end of the world!

 Don't go overboard on the alcohol: Make the wine a spritzer by mixing it with soda or sparkling water. It will help to keep your calories at bay and you'll also drink less.

 Treat yourself but don't lose control: You are allowed to let go a little, but keep it at bay. It's easy to forget about your willpower and self-control when you are away; however, limit yourself to one treat and not three!

 Don't skip meals to 'store up' calories: You know by now that it doesn't work that way. Eat your three meals a day and do your best to maintain a healthy balance of fruit, vegetables and protein.

Enjoying a night out

Most of us love a good night out in our favourite restaurant with a big glass of wine and great company. I know I do, anyway! When I began my journey I was definitely a bit apprehensive about eating out and feared I wouldn't enjoy it in the same way. For a start, there's always the confusion about what you should be avoiding and what you should be choosing. While I do relax a little at the weekends, I still try to go for the healthy option when I'm in a restaurant. When you are not cooking the food yourself, you have very little control over what actually goes into it. However, you can educate yourself about what the healthy choices are. Life doesn't stop just because you are trying to be healthy. In fact, it's quite the opposite. The best advice I can give you is to get out there, keep living and don't stop eating out! Here are my top tips for your restaurant visits.

 Before eating out, go on the restaurant's website and have a quick look at the menu. If you are prepared, you are less likely to make the wrong food choices.

Most restaurants have caught up with the ever-increasing demand for nutritious food and as a result are offering more variety in this area. Scan the menu for what you think are the healthy options. Don't always go for the same thing. To keep enjoying your food, you must have variety in your diet. Feel free to ask the waiter questions. They are obliged to give you information about the food you are ordering. How is it cooked, for example? You know yourself that you would rather it was grilled than fried. Don't be afraid to get what you want – you are the paying customer after all!

 Instead of potatoes or fries on the side, ask for salad or vegetables. Many restaurants provide very small portions of veg, so if you'd like more go ahead and ask. The good thing about vegetables is that they really fill you up, so you won't be desperate for carbs!

 Choose the fish. I usually do this when I'm out for a meal because I know it's good for me. It also works well with a side salad or vegetables, so you can't go wrong.

 Don't forget the water. There is nothing to say that you can't maintain your good habits when you're eating out. Water fills you up and stops you from going overboard on the wine!

 You don't have to finish everything on your plate. There is nobody standing over you, forcing you to eat everything. If you feel full, put down your knife and fork and take a break. People are far more likely to overeat when they are in a restaurant because they feel it's wrong to leave food. In future, ask the restaurant to put any leftovers in a box for you to take home.

If you have a sweet tooth that needs to be satisfied, share a pudding with somebody else. You'll get the same great taste but with half the calories, so it's a win, win, win! Sorbets are a great low-fat dessert and still taste good. Otherwise go for a coffee to round off your meal.

Dear stress, let's break up!

Dealing with stress

Each and every one of us deals with stress in a different way. Some of us can just address a situation and handle it as it happens. For others, it just seems too big and trying to cope becomes too much. Whatever category you fall into, we have all felt stressed at some point. When changes are occurring in our life, there is always the possibility that a level of stress could creep in and begin to make things difficult. Changing your lifestyle isn't easy and there will be moments when the journey seems incredibly tough. When I think back on my own journey, I can distinctly remember feeling frustrated when the weight didn't seem to be coming off as quickly as I would have liked. That in itself definitely brought about a level of stress.

If you are starting to feel the pressure, there are plenty of things you can do to help alleviate some of the stress:

Don't take too much on: Some people take the weight of the world on their shoulders, say 'yes' to everything and never get a minute to themselves. Now, more than ever, you need time that is quite simply just for 'you'. You do not need to be constantly running around without a moment to think. Your new lifestyle has meant many changes for you day-to-day, so try to put yourself first whenever possible. You don't have to be the one who is in control of absolutely everything.

Make lists: I think it's so important to have to-do lists, which allow you to see exactly what you have to get done. Writing a list alleviates the worry of having too many things in your head, which can be really overwhelming. Make life easier for yourself by getting a small notebook and start making lists!

Spend time with people you love: Friends and family are the ones who make us feel good about ourselves. They can make us laugh, give support and often share our burdens. To keep stress at bay, surround yourself with people who help you feel good about yourself. Make time for others if you are not doing this already. Even if it's with your partner, it's important you do this. Paul and I sit down for a meal together, just the two of us, during the week. We chat, laugh and share our news. This is a really healthy way of dealing with whatever is going on in our life.

 Write it down: Keeping a diary and writing down how you feel is a great way of keeping track of your emotions. It's also a form of therapy, as once you write things down you are often more able to let them go. Every day will provide new challenges. Putting pen to paper will enable you to track your progress, so when you look back you'll be able to see just how much you have achieved.

 Take breaks: You are not invincible and you can't keep going without the effects starting to show. You need to take a break, whether it is from work or home-life. Whatever your situation, learn how to take time out and look after you. Grab a coffee and read a magazine or go for a quick walk.

Doing everything right and you're still overweight?

It's a horrible feeling when you realise that, even though you think you've done everything right, you still haven't made progress. You've gone to the trouble of changing your eating habits, you've started exercising and you've tried to stay positive, and yet still nothing! Do not despair because there could be a reason why your weight-loss attempts haven't worked. Here are some possible explanations:

> *There could be a reason why your weight-loss attempts haven't worked.*

Watch your portion control and do not go overboard.

 You are still overeating. Just because you have begun eating healthier meals it doesn't mean you can eat more. Everything in moderation still applies with food – you can still clock up the calories and pile on the pounds if you eat too many nuts! Watch your portion control and do not go overboard.

 You are not eating breakfast. Skipping the most important meal of the day has the opposite effect of what you need to achieve – results. When you skip a meal you slow down your metabolism and, at the start of the day, this is not a good move. Even if you don't feel hungry, it's still important to eat something early in the morning.

 You're not eating enough 'real' foods. Perhaps you have changed your habits, but maybe you are still not including enough food in its natural form? Even if you are consuming fewer calories, if you're eating processed food you will struggle to see results. Make sure you're getting enough fruit, vegetables, lean meat and fish.

 You're fooling yourself into thinking you are eating healthily. It's actually really easy to convince ourselves that we are doing everything we should be, but if our clothes are still too tight something is wrong. Eating well and exercising doesn't come easily to everyone. If you are serious about losing weight, take the lifestyle choice seriously. You are the only person who can be in control of that. Decide today to make a change.

 You are not getting enough sleep. If you don't get at least seven hours of sleep every night, you won't focus properly the next day. Your instinct will be to go for carbs or sugar-filled foods to give you energy. Train yourself to get into the habit of getting a proper rest every night (see page 67).

You're still eating white bread. Sorry to disappoint you, ladies, but if you want to get on the road to a slimmer stomach, you have to ban white bread from your diet. Aside from the fact that it has little nutritional value, it is a refined carb and therefore a recipe for disaster. Switch to wholegrain once and for all! I eat McCambridge brown bread and limit myself to two slices on Saturday and Sunday. Remember: if it's white, don't bite!

 You're not exercising right. Whatever form of exercise you have decided to take up might not be producing the results you had hoped for. If possible, when you are starting out, seek some kind of professional advice in terms of what you should and shouldn't be doing. This way, you can make sure that all your hard work is not being done in vain.

 You're not concentrating when you do eat. Eating in front of the television, whilst on your laptop or at your desk are all bad ideas. They lead to you eating fast and eating too much. You need to give your meal times your full attention in order to ensure that you don't fall into either of these traps. Make time for food, avoid distractions and keep your mind on the task in hand! Sit down, eat slowly and practise putting your knife and fork down between bites.

 Cut out the stress. Whatever it is that causes stress in your life, find a way of reducing it. It is one of the things that will prevent you from shifting the pounds. When we feel over-stressed we are more likely to seek comfort from food and also we find it harder to stay motivated.

You are looking for a quick fix. Like I say time and time again, there is no such thing. If you want to lose weight, and keep it off, it is going to take time. Accept that and you will be more likely to succeed.

If you want to lose weight, and keep it off, it is going to take time.

Afterword

Embrace it – losing weight means a whole new wardrobe! There is something about losing weight that makes the prospect of clothes shopping an incredibly exciting experience and I hope that this is something that you are starting to appreciate. As your weight falls off, you begin to gain confidence and start to believe in yourself. Isn't it the best feeling in the world to recognise you have achieved something you never thought was possible? The feeling you get when you start to explore fashion is amazing! I say this both as a woman who has been in your position and as a stylist. The change I have seen in some of the women I work with is incredible. It's as if they have discovered something brand new about themselves and that is brilliant.

You can use this newfound confidence as an incentive to continue your hard work. It's fun to go shopping for clothes that make you look and feel good. Suddenly you find you can experiment more with colour; no longer does black have to be your wardrobe staple. I'm not saying get rid of all the black clothes in your wardrobe; just try to explore different shades and styles. Be more adventurous in your choices and pick up clothes you would never have imagined yourself wearing. You don't have to follow every single fashion trend out there – just find what works for you. Your clothes should enhance your newfound confidence. Take a friend shopping with you or enjoy time on your own, but try to embrace the experience.

The other tip that I want to give you as you begin to lose weight is to learn to let go. By letting go I mean getting rid of your fat clothes. If they don't fit you any more, why keep them? Give them away to the local charity shop. You have made a decision to change your lifestyle, and that doesn't involve going backwards, so they are part of your past. Holding onto them is like a security blanket, which you don't need – you are going forwards, not backwards, from now on. Stay focused and excited about what lies ahead. Be proud of what you have achieved and celebrate it. You now have the opportunity to reinvent yourself.

Index

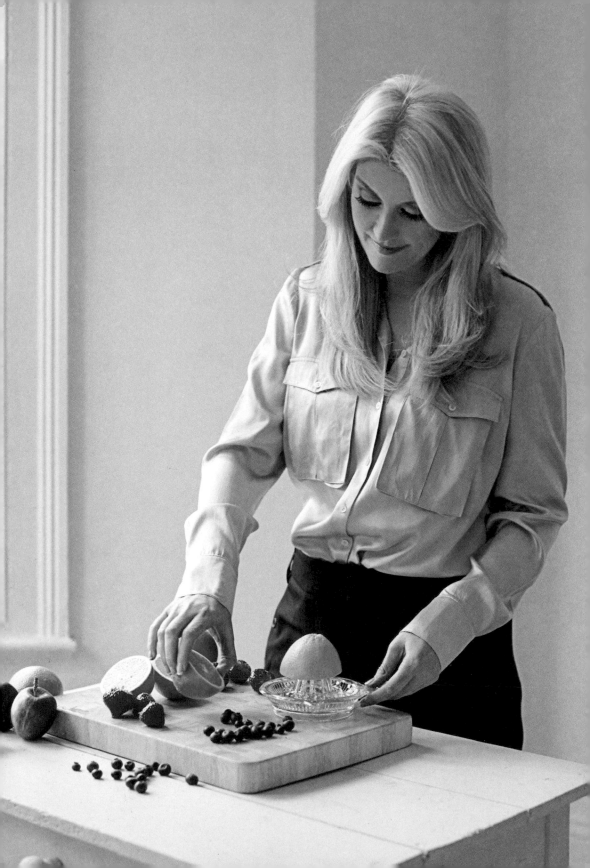